Artificial Intelligence for the Internet of Health Things

Biomedical and Robotics Healthcare

Series Editors:
Utku Kose, Jude Hemanth, Omer Deperlioglu

Artificial Intelligence for the Internet of Health Things
Deepak Gupta, Eswaran Perumal, and K. Shankar

Biomedical Signal and Image Examination with Entropy-Based Techniques
V. Rajinikanth, K. Kamalanand, C. Emmanuel, and B. Thayumanavan

Mechano-Electric Correlations in the Human Physiological System
A. Bakiya, K. Kamalanand and, R. L. J. De Britto

For more information about this series, please visit: https://www.routledge.com/
Biomedical-and-Robotics-Healthcare/book-series/BRHC

Artificial Intelligence for the Internet of Health Things

K. Shankar, Eswaran Perumal, Deepak Gupta

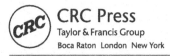

CRC Press
Taylor & Francis Group
Boca Raton London New York

CRC Press is an imprint of the
Taylor & Francis Group, an **informa** business

MATLAB® is a trademark of The MathWorks, Inc. and is used with permission. The MathWorks does not warrant the accuracy of the text or exercises in this book. This book's use or discussion of MATLAB® software or related products does not constitute endorsement or sponsorship by The MathWorks of a particular pedagogical approach or particular use of the MATLAB® software.

First edition published 2021
by CRC Press
6000 Broken Sound Parkway NW, Suite 300, Boca Raton, FL 33487-2742
and by CRC Press
2 Park Square, Milton Park, Abingdon, Oxon, OX14 4RN

© 2021 Taylor & Francis Group, LLC
CRC Press is an imprint of Taylor & Francis Group, LLC

The right of K. Shankar, Eswaran Perumal, and Deepak Gupta to be identified as authors of this work has been asserted by them in accordance with sections 77 and 78 of the Copyright, Designs and Patents Act 1988.

ISBN: 978-0-367-74497-7 (hbk)
ISBN: 978-1-003-15909-4 (ebk)

Typeset in Times LT Std
by KnowledgeWorks Global Ltd.

Contents

Author Biographies

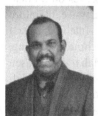

K. Shankar (Member, IEEE) is currently a Postdoctoral Fellow with the Department of Computer Applications, Alagappa University, Karaikudi, India. He has authored/coauthored 65+ ISI journal articles (with total Impact Factor 200+) and more than 100 Scopus indexed articles. He has authored/edited conference proceedings, book chapters, and three books published by Springer. He has been a part of various seminars, paper presentations, research paper reviews, and convener and a session chair of several conferences. He has displayed vast success in continuously acquiring new knowledge and applying innovative pedagogies and has always aimed to be an effective educator and have a global outlook. His current research interests include healthcare applications, secret image sharing scheme, digital image security, cryptography, the Internet of Things, and optimization algorithms. He has guest-edited several special issues at many journals published by SAGE, TechScience, Inderscience, and MDPI. He has served as a Guest Editor and an Associate Editor in SCI, Scopus indexed journals, such as Elsevier, Springer, IGI, Wiley, and MDPI. He has served as a chair (program, publications, technical committee, and track) on several international conferences. He has delivered several invited and keynote talks, and reviewed technology-leading articles for journals such as *Scientific Reports-Nature, IEEE Transactions on Neural Networks and Learning Systems, IEEE Journal of Biomedical and Health Informatics, IEEE Transactions on Reliability, IEEE Access*, and *IEEE Internet of Things*.

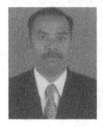

Eswaran Perumal received an MSc degree in Computer Science and Information Technology from Madurai Kamaraj University, India, in 2003, and received an MTech. and a PhD. degree in Computer and Information Technology from Manonmaniam Sundaranar University, India, in 2005 and 2010, respectively. In 2010, he joined the Department of Computer Science and Engineering, PSN College of Engineering and Technology, as Assistant Professor. Since May 2012, he has been with the Department of Computer Science and Engineering, Alagappa University, Karaikudi, India, as Assistant Professor. He was the recipient of the Junior Research Fellowship Award of the University Grants Commission, New Delhi, in 2008. He has published more than 35 scientific papers in the field of Digital Image Processing and Data Mining. His research interests include Digital Image Processing, focusing on Color Image Edge Detection, Data Mining, and Computer and Communication Networks.

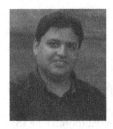 **Dr. Deepak Gupta** is an eminent academician who plays versatile roles and responsibilities juggling between lectures, research, publications, consultancy, community service, PhD, and post-doctorate supervision. With 12 years of rich expertise in teaching and 2 years in industry, he focuses on rational and practical learning. He has contributed massive literature in the fields of Human-Computer Interaction, Intelligent Data Analysis, Nature-Inspired Computing, Machine Learning, and Soft Computing. He is working as Assistant Professor at Maharaja Agrasen Institute of Technology (GGSIPU), Delhi, India. He has served as Editor-in-Chief, Guest Editor, Associate Editor in SCI, and various other reputed journals (Elsevier, Springer, Wiley, and MDPI). He has actively been part of various reputed international conferences. He is not only backed with a strong profile but his innovative ideas, research's end-results, and notion of implementation of technology in the medical field is by and large contributing to the society significantly. He is currently a Post-Doc researcher at University of Valladolid, Spain. He has completed his first Post-Doc from Inatel, Brazil, and PhD from Dr. APJ Abdul Kalam Technical University. He has authored/edited 33 books with national/international level publishers (Elsevier, Springer, Wiley, Katson). He has published 101 scientific research publications in reputed international journals and conferences including 49 SCI indexed journals of IEEE, Elsevier, Springer, Wiley, and many more. He is Editor-in-Chief of *OA Journal-Computers*; Associate Editor of *Expert Systems* (Wiley), *Intelligent Decision Technologies* (IOS Press), and *Journal of Computational and Theoretical Nenoscience*; and Honorary Editor of *ICSES Transactions on Image Processing and Pattern Recognition*. He is also a series editor of "Smart Sensors Technology for BioMedical Engineering" (Elsevier), "Intelligent Biomedical Data Analysis" (De Gruyter, Germany), and "Computational Intelligence for Data Analysis" (Bentham Science). He is also associated with various professional bodies such as ISTE, IAENG, IACSIT, SCIEI, ICSES, UACEE, Internet Society, SMEI, IAOP, and IAOIP and invited as a Faculty Resource Person/Session Chair/Reviewer/TPC member in different FDP, conferences, and journals. He is the convener of the "ICICC" conference series.

Preface

Artificial intelligence (AI) techniques have the capability of transforming the way that doctors handle patients and deliver services. The AI techniques can help doctors by offering updated medical information to provide effective patient care. The Internet of Things (IoT) refers to sensing devices linked to one another through the Internet. IoT devices can be embed into the healthcare sector to derive Internet of Health Things (IoHT) for patient monitoring through wearables, smart sensors, and smartphones. IoHT tools assist doctors to observe patients in remote areas. Designing AI techniques with IoHT will be key for smart hospitals to improve healthcare applications and services.

This book, *Artificial Intelligence for the Internet of Health Things,* covers recent developments in the field of AI and IoHT, particularly for the healthcare sector. It offers a detailed explanation of the basic concepts, design issues, and research results of AI in the IoHT sector. The effective integration of AI and IoT in the healthcare sector avoids unplanned downtime, improves operating efficiency, enables new products and services, and increases risk management. It is an invaluable resource giving knowledge on the core and specialized issues in the field, making it highly suitable for both new and experienced researchers in this field. The works submitted within the scope of this book can be organized into 15 chapters, and the topics include AI, IoT, and cloud computing (CC)–enabled medical diagnosis of different diseases such as diabetic retinopathy, diabetes mellitus, brain tumor, skin lesions, hemorrhage detection, breast cancer, and heart disease.

In the following, selected papers are briefed based on their core topic.

- Chapter 1 offers an introductory overview of AI techniques, a brief history of AI in healthcare, and different types of AI devices for clinical data generation. The chapter also explains the different application perspectives of AI techniques in the healthcare sector.
- Chapter 2 introduces the role of IoT and CC in the medical field including the fundamental framework, CC concepts, components in IoT-based healthcare systems, and different IoT-based healthcare applications.
- Chapter 3 provides a brief discussion of wearable technologies. Also, the issues that exist in the design and utilization of wearables are neatly listed. It also aims to explain the different application perspective of wearables on medical diagnosis.
- Chapter 4 proposes an IoT and cloud-based disease diagnosis model using Particle Swarm Optimization with Artificial Neural Networks. The proposed method is used to monitor the diagnosis of the presence of diabetes diseases and their severity level.
- Chapter 5 presents an IoT-based Improved Grey Optimization with Support Vector Machine for gastrointestinal hemorrhage detection and diagnosis model. The proposed model aims to determine patterns and bleeding regions in Wireless Capsule Endoscopy (WCE) images.

- Chapter 6 develops an effective Personalized Medicine Recommendation System using an Ensemble of Extreme Learning Machine (ELM) Model. The presented model recommends drugs to patients according to medical diagnosis data.
- Chapter 7 introduces a novel Map Reduce-Based Hybrid Decision Tree with TFIDF Algorithm for Public Sentiment Mining of Diabetes Mellitus. The proposed method is applied for classifying information depending upon the polarities of every context in social network data.
- Chapter 8 devises a new IoT-based Breast Cancer Diagnosis using Hybrid Feature Extraction with an Optimal Support Vector Machine–based Classification Model.
- Chapter 9 aims to develop a new Deep Neural Network (DNN) with Directional Local Ternary Quantized Extrema Patterns (DLTerQEPs) and a Crest Line Technique for Cloud-Based Medical Image Retrieval model.
- Chapter 10 introduces IoHT with Cloud-Based Brain Tumor Detection using Particle Swarm Optimization with Support Vector Machine. The PSO-SVM classifier model is applied for the classification of BT images as benign or malign.
- Chapter 11 develops an AI-Based Hough Transform with Adaptive Neuro-Fuzzy Inference System (ANFIS) for a Diabetic Retinopathy Classification Model. The ANFIS model detects and classifies the retinal fundus image into different levels of severity.
- Chapter 12 proposes an IoHT-Enabled Intelligent Skin Lesion Detection and Classification Model in Dermoscopic Images. The proposed method makes use of the SVM model and is applied to classify the set of dermoscopic images into appropriate classes.
- Chapter 13 devises an IoHT-based image compression model using the Modified Cuckoo Search (MCS) Algorithm with Vector Quantization. The MCS is an extension of the classical cuckoo search algorithm (CSA) by modifying the intensification and diversification models.
- Chapter 14 devises an improved particle swarm optimization (IPSO) algorithm with a discrete wavelet transform (DWT) for secure medical image transmission. The proposed IPSO-DWT algorithm aims to select optimal pixels for embedding secret images.
- Finally, Chapter 15 develops an IoHT with wearable devices–based feature extraction and a deep neural networks classification model for heart disease diagnosis.

1 Artificial Intelligence (AI) for IoHT – An Introduction

1.1 ARTIFICIAL INTELLIGENCE (AI) IN THE HEALTHCARE DOMAIN

Presently, there is a need for a model with its linked gadgets, persons, and networks completely integrated on the Internet of Health Things (IoHT), which offers medicinal services to patients, monitoring patients, and offering drug recommendations. The IoHT incorporates both technological expertise and electronics. Artificial intelligence (AI) is the application of science-based research and the development of smart machines. The people without the knowledge of intelligent machines conjure images of charismatic human-based systems and robots, as depicted in science fiction [1]. The most familiar media reports of applying aerial surveillance drones, driverless cars, and other features of perils in emerging smart machines, which has been improved with common awareness. AI models and approaches are predefined from other formulations. Several domains of AI schemes are available in the literature [2].

AI models are applied in automobiles, aircraft guidance fields, smartphone equipment like audio analysis applications such as Apple's Siri, Internet web browsers, and a plethora of alternate practical actions. AI methodologies tend to resolve problems and perform events in stable, effective, and productive types when compared with other possibilities. The nature of mental healthcare domains provides the merits and advancements in AI [3]. For instance, processing models to learning, understanding, and reasoning helps the experts in clinical decision-making, analysis, diagnostics, and so on. AI approaches could be more advanced in self-care devices to enhance people's lifestyles, such as communicative mobile health fields that know the patterns as well as priorities of customers. AI results in the enhancement of public health under the assistance of detecting health risks and data inventions. An alternate instance of AI is that virtual humans are capable of communicating with care seekers and can give appropriate remedies to cure the disease. This chapter depicts the chance of applying AI models and methods for healthcare operations in future advancements [4, 5].

The main objective of AI is to develop machines with the potential to perform tasks such as essential intelligence, like reasoning, learning, planning, problem resolving, as well as perception. The relevant fields involved in AI are shown in Fig. 1.1. This domain was named by computer scientist John McCarty, and Marvin Minsky, Nathan Rochester, and Claude Shannon implied it at the Dartmouth Conference. The key objective of this conference was to set a novel domain of science that contributes to the study of modern devices. Each perception of learning intelligence could be so precisely defined that a machine is made to develop it. At

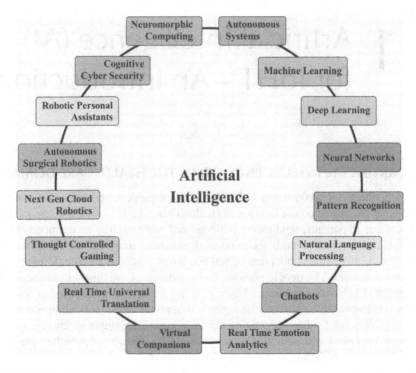

FIGURE 1.1 Relevant fields of AI.

the time of the conference, Allen Newell, J.C. Shaw, and Herbert Simon illustrated the Logic Theorist (LT), as the initial computer program manufactured to reflect problem resolving techniques [6].

In the last few decades, AI has been developed into multidisciplinary fields with computer science, engineering, psychology, and so on. Few objectives can be accomplished by the application of AI, to develop a framework to achieve remarkable events such as computer vision, audio recognition, and detection of patterns that exist in data [7]. It mainly concentrates on specialized intelligent actions that have been named as Weak AI, also termed as Applied AI. Instead of thinking that humans can play chess, Deep Blue employs the application of brute force approaches to estimate the possibilities to compute the offensive as well as defensive movements. The term "Strong AI" was coined by philosopher John Searle in 1980, and defines the aim of deploying machines with common AI. The major intention of Strong AI is to deploy machines with smart capability that is indistinguishable from humans. Such resources are typically narrow and accurate tasks, namely the function of arithmetic task. AI is utilized to invent the intelligent nature of machines to perform the events of human behavior. AI might be the form of either hardware or software that can stand alone, distributed over the computer networks, or embedded into a robot. Besides, it is in the form of intelligent and independent agents that are capable of communicating with the corresponding platform in the decision-making process. AI is combined with biological operations for brain computer interfaces

(BCIs), which is manufactured with biological objectives (biological AI), and small molecular structures referred to as nanotechnology [8].

Several clinical decision support systems (CDSSs) were presented by the use of AI approaches and finds useful in several domains [9]. This chapter offers an introductory explanation of AI concepts, evolution, clinical data generation, and AI techniques in healthcare. This chapter also discusses several applications of AI techniques developed in the healthcare sector.

1.2 EVOLUTION OF AI IN THE MEDICAL SECTOR

Rule-based methods achieved most of the success in the 1970s, which includes interpreting electrocardiograms (ECGs), diagnosing diseases, selecting proper remedies, offering the interpretations of clinical reasoning, and helping doctors in producing diagnostic statements for severe patients. Therefore, rule-based systems are the most expensive to develop and can also be vulnerable since they need explicit presentations of decision rules as well as human-relied updates. Additionally, it is very complex to encode higher-order communications between various pieces of knowledge provided by diverse professionals, and the working function of systems is reduced by an extensive advancement of medical knowledge. Therefore, it is very hard to execute a system that incorporates the deterministic as well as probabilistic reasoning to narrow down the related clinical content, prefer the diagnostic statement, and advanced therapy [10].

In contrast to the first generation of AI, which is based on the advice of medical experts and a formulation of effective decision rules, current AI studies have alleviated machine learning (ML) techniques, which consider the difficult interactions to discover the patterns that exist in data. Based on the types of functions that have been induced to resolve, fundamental ML techniques were classified into two classes: supervised and unsupervised [11]. The supervised ML approach was operated by gathering a large number of "training" cases that were comprised with inputs like fundus images and target output labels such as existence or lack of diabetic retinopathy (DR). By the pattern recognition of labeled input and output pairs, the method attempts to generate specific output for the provided input. Also, it has been developed for identifying the best parameters to reduce the deviations among the predictions for training cases and monitored results. The generalizability of a method could be evaluated under the application of the test set. Classification, regression, and characterization of similarity between instances of the same results are vastly applied functions of supervised ML techniques.

Unsupervised learning acquires basic patterns from unlabeled data to discover subclusters of actual data, to find outliers of data, and generate low-dimensional presentations of data. It is pointed out that the discovery of minimum dimension representations for labeled instances has to be more efficient to attain a supervised model. Here, ML approaches tend to develop the AI domains that have been served as the discovery of existing unknown patterns in data with no requirement of particular decision rules for every specific task that assumes for difficult communications between the input features. ML has been one of the applied systems to deploy AI units.

Several types of intelligent neural networks (NNs) are comprised of a maximum number of layers. NNs have a massive number of layers capable of modeling tedious relations from input and output where it requires more data, processing duration, and latest structural designs to reach optimized functions. Various layers, numerical tasks for neurons, and regularizing models were deployed. For instance, convolutional layers are more helpful for extracting spatial or temporal relations, while recurrent layers apply circular links to design the temporal actions. Besides, diverse types of initialization and activation functions are used in improving the method's function. The integration of such units activates the NN to manage multiple inputs with and without spatial or temporal basis. A smart NN could be constrained with a higher number of attributes and consume large computational resources for training purposes.

The improvising application of electronic health record (EHR) systems is comprised of a set of large-scale medicinal data and enables a smooth combination of AI models as a clinical workflow (Fig. 1.2). Traditionally, medical experts gather the medical data from patients to make a clinical decision and save the reports and treatment plans as health records (Fig. 1.2a). The decision support system (DSS) gathers the medical-related data to provide suggestions for doctors (Fig. 1.2b). There are several methods to combine the DSS into the clinical workflow; for example, the DSS is capable of collecting data from patients and EHRs, provides suggestions to physicians, and archives in a system output of EHRs (Fig. 1.2c). Several approaches are associated with complete automatic clinical systems, such as the independent tools gather data from patients to make decisions and produce the outcome into EHRs (Fig. 1.2d). Data from EHR models give brief data regarding patients, such as medicinal notes as well as laboratory measures, activating the field of natural language processing (NLP) approaches to obtain codified vocabularies [12].

1.3 USE OF AI DEVICES FOR CLINICAL DATA GENERATION

Before the existence of an AI system in a healthcare field, it has to undergo training with the help of data produced from clinical events, such as screening, diagnosis, treatment schedule, and so on; thus, it can acquire the data from the same set of subjects, correlations among subject features, as well as results of interest. Such clinical data does not exist in a reduced form of demographics, medical notes, digital values from medical gadgets, external observations, as well as clinical laboratory and images. In a diagnosis phase, a substantial portion of AI research examines the data from diagnosis imaging, genetic testing, as well as electro-diagnosis.

Here, AI tools are divided into two main classes. In the case of medical domains, the ML strategy tries to collect the patient's details. The latter class is associated with NLP approaches, which obtain data from unstructured data such as clinical notes to provide enriched structured medicinal information. The NLP procedures aim at changing the texts to a machine-readable format that is screened using ML approaches. The flowchart in Fig. 1.3 defines the road map from clinical data, by NLP data enrichment, as well as ML data investigation to make decisions. The road map has been initiated and concluded with clinical events. If the AI models are robust, it is inspired by the clinical issues and used in clinical practice.

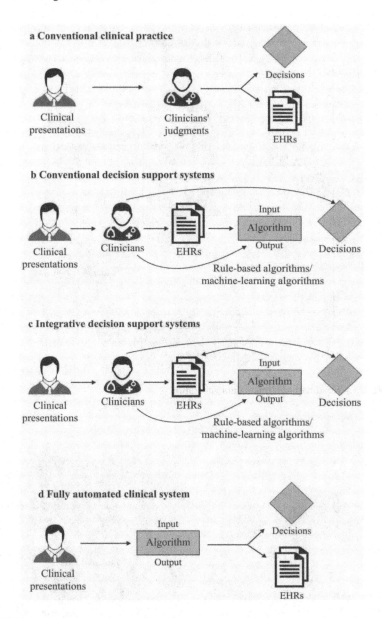

FIGURE 1.2 Flow of information in healthcare.

1.4 TYPES OF AI OF RELEVANCE TO HEALTHCARE

AI is one of the models that consists of a few other techniques, namely ML and deep learning (DL) as shown in Fig. 1.4. These methodologies are related to the adverse effect of the healthcare domain; however, a specialized task is vastly supported [13]. Some models of AI methods are highly significant to healthcare, as explained in this section.

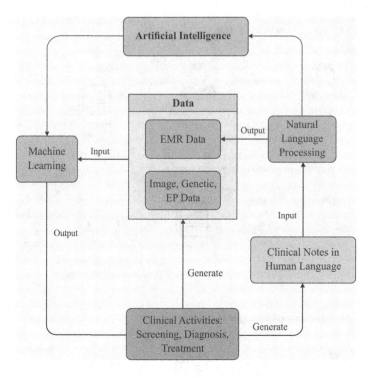

FIGURE 1.3   Roadmap of clinical data generation.

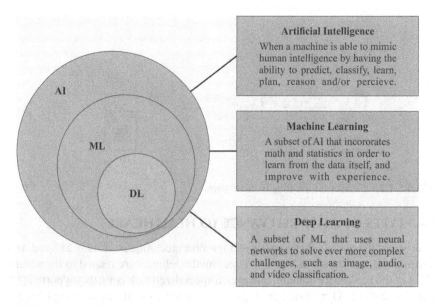

FIGURE 1.4   AI, ML, and DL models.

1.4.1 MACHINE LEARNING – NEURAL NETWORKS AND DEEP LEARNING

In this model, ML is known to be a statistical approach that is applied for fitting techniques to data by training schemes along with data. ML is one of the typical forms of approach in AI; in a Deloitte survey presented by United States managers pursuing AI, 63% of organizations applied ML in the business process [14]. It is known to be a wider approach along with AI and several models.

A greater majority of ML and accurate medicine fields acquire a training data set where the outcome variable is predefined, which is named as supervised learning. A tedious ML is called an NN, in which the model is accessible in healthcare research that is utilized in classifying applications such as climate analysis, where a patient requires the desired data. Concerning inputs and outputs, weights of the feature correlate with the inputs with outputs. In addition, it tends to the neurons' processing signals; however, the analogy of the brain's performance is comparatively vulnerable. The tedious form of ML is involved in DL, or NN approaches, with massive levels of features that detect the simulation outcomes. Several hidden models are uncovered by the rapid computation of current graphics processing units (GPUs) and cloud structures.

A general domain of DL in healthcare is the analysis of cancerous lesions in radiology images. DL has been widely used in radionics, the forecasting of medically related variables in imaging data across the human eye. These radionics, as well as DL, are often applied in oncology-oriented image detection. Such integration tends to improve the accuracy in diagnosing an existing production of automatic tools for image analysis, called computer-aided detection (CAD). In addition, DL is an increased application for audio analysis and the NLP, defined in the next section. In contrary to statistical analysis, every feature in a DL approach has a human observer. Finally, the definition of the model's results might be complex for interpretation.

1.4.2 NATURAL LANGUAGE PROCESSING

Sensing the human language is the main aim of AI developers. Hence, NLP contains applications such as audio analysis, text investigation, translation, and alternate goals relevant to the language [15]. It is comprised of two fundamental models: statistical and semantic NLP. Statistical NLP depends upon ML and it involves the current improvement of accuracy of recognition. It needs a massive "corpus" or body of language to learn. The leading applications of NLP are the development, learning, and classification of clinical documents and published studies. NLP is capable of examining the unstructured clinical notes on patients, and patient communications, as well as carrying out the AI conversation.

1.4.3 RULE-BASED EXPERT SYSTEMS

Expert systems depend upon the set of "if-then" rules that are the dominant model for AI and widely used in later periods. The CDSS model was vastly used across the world. Several EHR models offer a furnished collection of rules along with systems today [16]. Expert systems require human professionals as well as knowledge engineers to create a sequence of rules in specific applications. It performs quite well to a point and is simple in understanding. Therefore, when a knowledge domain modifies, the rules might be complex and time-consuming. Also, it is being slowly replaced in healthcare with the application of several techniques that depend upon data and ML algorithms.

1.4.4 PHYSICAL ROBOTS

Physical robots are the most popular and used of around 200,000 industrial robots that have been deployed globally. A physical robot performs predetermined operations such as lifting, relocation, welding, and assembling of objects in places such as firms and warehouses [17], and providing supplies. The robots collaborate with humans trained easily under the movement of the desired operation. They are very intelligent, while AI abilities are incorporated in "brains" as operating systems (OSs). Surgical robots were accepted in the United States in 2000. These robots offer superpowers by boosting visual activities, creating precise and lower invasive incisions, stitching wounds, and so on. The most significant decisions are still made by human surgeons.

1.4.5 ROBOTIC PROCESS AUTOMATION

This is used to perform the structured digital tasks in administrative applications in which a human user applies the script or rules. Among other forms of AI, it is cheaper and easier to program and has more visible events. Robotic process automation (RPA) does not contribute to the robots and computer programs on servers. It is based on an integration of workflow, business rules, and the "presentation layer" combination with information systems to be treated as a semi-intelligent user. In healthcare, it has been applied for repeated tasks such as prior authentication and extending patient billing.

1.5 AI-BASED APPLICATIONS IN HEALTHCARE

Diagnosis, as well as remedy of disease, mainly focuses on AI, while the MYCIN AI program was deployed at Stanford to analyze blood-borne bacterial infections. It is primary rule-based systems that depict accurate diagnosing as well as treating disease, where it has not been used in clinical practice. Substantially, it is better when compared with human experts and poorly combined with physician workflows and medical record systems. In recent times, IBM's Watson has obtained reasonable attention in the media for precision medicine, specifically cancer diagnosis as well as remedies [18].

Implementation problems with AI may be more complex in healthcare firms. The rule-based systems are combined inside EHR systems in the National Health Service (NHS). Rule-based CDSSs are complex for maintaining medical knowledge variations and cannot be managed with the explosion of data as well as knowledge relied on genomic, proteomic, metabolic, and alternate "omic-based" models to care. It has been a changing one, which has been present in research labs and tech firms, instead of clinical practice. Such findings are relied on radiological image analysis; although few others contribute to alternate types of images such as retinal scanning or genomic-specified precision medicine.

The findings depend upon statistically-based ML methods and ensuring that the evidence and probability-based treatment has been regarded as positive, which has challenges in medical ethics. Tech firms, as well as start-ups, are assiduously on similar problems. Google, for instance, uses the collaboration of health delivery systems to create predictive methods from big data to warn the doctor's high-risk status, like sepsis and heart failure. Google, Enlitic, and diverse start-ups are developing AI-based image interpretation techniques. Jvion provides a clinical success machine that finds the patients who are most at risk and responds to the treatment protocols. It is comprised of massive firms that concentrate on diagnosis as well as treatment recommendations for finite cancers relied on genetic profiles. As many cancers are comprised of a genetic basis, human experts are increasingly tedious to find every genetic variant of cancer and response for novel drugs as well as protocols. Organizations such as Foundation Medicine and Flatiron Health, owned by Roche, specialize in this model. Such techniques are efficient in detection, although it lacks related data that consists of predictive capability, such as patient socioeconomic conditions. The combination of issues tends to be a greater obstacle to extensive execution of AI, which cannot offer accurate as well as productive recommendations, and several AI-relied abilities for diagnosing and treatment from tech firms are supportive in nature of care. Few EHR vendors have been initiated to combine the reduced AI events into offerings. Providers are substantially combined until EHR vendors include maximum AI abilities.

1.5.1 PATIENT ENGAGEMENT AND ADHERENCE APPLICATIONS

Patient engagement and adherence are known to be a last-mile problem of healthcare and the final obstacle among impractical as well as good health results; the application, economical results, as well as member experience. Such factors were reported by the application of big data and AI. Providers and hospitals employ clinical expertise to create a plan of care that enhances the chronic or acute patient's health. Therefore, it doesn't matter when a patient fails to develop behavioral adjustment, for example, weight loss, allocation of follow-up visits, or occupying the prescriptions with a treatment plan [19]. Noncompliance is defined as if a patient cannot apply the treatment because there has been a major issue with the provided drugs. When a closer involvement by patients tends to provide an optimal result, the AI-based abilities are in personalizing and contextualizing with an emphasis on applying ML and business rules engines to stimulate the interventions with care continuum. Messaging alerts and related, desired content triggers events at moments that have promising research, through the data generated by provider EHR systems, biosensors, watches, smartphones, conversational interfaces, and alternate instrumentation, where the recommendations are tailored by relating patient details to alternate treatment fashion for the same cohorts.

1.5.2 ADMINISTRATIVE APPLICATIONS

This has been correlated with administrative domains in healthcare. The exploitation of AI has a minimum potential revolution when related to patient care; however, it is capable of providing substantial objectives. Such requirements in healthcare are due to a nurse in the United States spending a maximum of 25% of their work time on regulatory as well as administrative events. It is employed in diverse applications of healthcare, such as claims events, clinical documentation, financial cycle management, as well as medical records management. Some healthcare firms are implemented with chatbots for patient communication, mental health and wellness, and telehealth. But, in a US survey of 500 people regarding 5 chatbots employed in healthcare, patients presented concerns regarding secret data, defining tedious health conditions and worst application. An alternate AI model with related claims and billing administration is ML, which is employed in the probabilistic mapping of data over diverse databases. Reliably identifying, examining, and correcting coding problems, as well as inaccurate claims, stores every stakeholder and health insurers, governments, and providers with maximum time, money, and effort. Ineffective claims that have slipped through the cracks constitute vital potential waiting to be unlocked under the application of data-matching and claiming audits.

1.5.3 IMPLICATIONS FOR THE HEALTHCARE WORKFORCE

Here, it is associated with reasonable focus that AI leads to automated jobs and substantial replacement of the workforce. A Deloitte collaboration with the Oxford Martin Institute deployed that 35% of UK jobs can be automatic by using AI. Alternate studies show that if some automated jobs are feasible, varied external factors rather than the model can reduce the job loss, such as the expense of automated methods, labor market growth and cost, merits of automatic simple labor replacement, and regulator social approval. Such factors limit the actual job loss of minimum value. The reduced incursion of AI with industry and a complex combination of AI to clinical workflows as well as EHR systems are responsible for the absence of job impact. It is the same in healthcare jobs that are automatic and involve dealing with electronic data, radiology, and pathology. Even though in jobs such as radiologist and pathologist, the induction of AI in these applications might be gradual. The models such as DL are more stable in diagnosing and classifying images; still, maximum issues remain in radiology jobs, where it does not appear rapidly.

Substantial variations are essential in medical regulation as well as health insurance for automatic image analysis. The same factors have been presented for pathology and alternate digitally based facts of medicine. Also, it has the viability of novel jobs that would be developed in AI models.

1.5.4 ETHICAL IMPLICATIONS

There are diverse ethical implementations in the application of AI in healthcare. Healthcare decisions have been uniquely created by humans for the last few decades, and the utilization of smart machines helps accountability, transparency, permission, and privacy issues. When the patient data is provided for cancer screening, the AI models will be used for inpatient analysis and recovery process. Also, ML in health-care might be subjected to algorithmic bias, rather detecting the higher likelihood of disease based on gender with causal factors. The effective and final approaches to impact human societies, it requires constant attention and thoughtful suggestion for several years.

1.6   CONCLUSION

In the last few decades, AI has been developed into multidisciplinary fields with computer science, engineering, psychology, philosophy, ethics, and so on. Several CDSSs were presented by the use of AI approaches and finds that are useful in several domains. This chapter has provided a brief overview of AI and its applicabil-ity in the medical domain. Besides, the historical overview of AI in the healthcare domain has been provided clearly. Along with that, a detailed description of the use of AI devices to generate clinical data of patients has been discussed. Moreover, different types of AI techniques in healthcare have been elaborated. Finally, sev-eral applications of AI techniques developed in the literature have been discussed comprehensively.

REFERENCES

[1] Rodrigues, J.J., Segundo, D.B.D.R., Junqueira, H.A., Sabino, M.H., Prince, R.M., Al-Muhtadi, J., and De Albuquerque, V.H.C. Enabling technologies for the Internet of Health Things. *IEEE Access*, 6, 13129–13141, 2018.

[2] Elhoseny, M., Shankar, K., and Uthayakumar, J. Intelligent diagnostic prediction and classification system for chronic kidney disease. *Scientific Reports*, 9 (1), 1–14, 2019.

[3] Eskofier, B.M., Lee, S.I., Baron, M., Simon, A., Martindale, C.F., Gaßner, H., and Klucken, J. An overview of smart shoes in the internet of health things: Gait and mobil-ity assessment in health promotion and disease monitoring. *Applied Sciences*, 7 (10), 986, 2017.

[4] Lakshmanaprabu, S. K., Mohanty, S. N., Krishnamoorthy, S., Uthayakumar, J., and Shankar, K. Online clinical decision support system using optimal deep neural net-works. *Applied Soft Computing*, 81, 105487, 2019.

[5] da Costa, C.A., Pasluosta, C.F., Eskofier, B., da Silva, D.B., and da Rosa Righi, R. Internet of Health Things: Toward intelligent vital signs monitoring in hospital wards. *Artificial Intelligence in Medicine*, 89, 61–69, 2018.

[6] Elhoseny, M., Bian, G. B., Lakshmanaprabu, S. K., Shankar, K., Singh, A. K., and Wu, W. Effective features to classify ovarian cancer data in internet of medical things. *Computer Networks*, 159, 147–156, 2019.

[7] Raj, R. J. S., Shobana, S. J., Pustokhina, I. V., Pustokhin, D. A., Gupta, D., and Shankar, K. Optimal feature selection-based medical image classification using deep learning model in Internet of Medical Things. *IEEE Access*, 8, 58006–58017, 2020.

[8] Lakshmanaprabu, S. K., Mohanty, S. N., Shankar, K., Arunkumar, N., and Ramirez, G. Optimal deep learning model for classification of lung cancer on CT images. *Future Generation Computer Systems*, 92, 374–382, 2019.

[9] Yu, K. H. et al. Predicting ovarian cancer patients' clinical response to platinum-based chemotherapy by their tumor proteomic signatures. *Journal of Proteome Research*, 15 (8), 2455–2465, 2016.

[10] Beam, A. L. and Kohane, I. S. Translating artificial intelligence into clinical care. *JAMA,* 316, 2368–2369, 2016.

[11] Ching, T. et al. Opportunities and obstacles for deep learning in biology and medicine. *Journal of Royal Society Interface,* 15, 20170387, 2018.

[12] van Ginneken, B., Setio, A. A., Jacobs, C. and Ciompi, F. Off-the-shelf convolutional neural network features for pulmonary nodule detection in computed tomography scans. In IEEE 12th International Symposium Biomedical Imaging (ISBI), 2015, 286–289.

[13] Jiang, F., Jiang, Y., Zhi, H., Dong, Y., Li, H., Ma, S., Wang, Y., Dong, Q., Shen, H., and Wang, Y. Artificial intelligence in healthcare: past, present and future. *Stroke and Vascular Neurology,* 2 (4), 230–243, 2017.

[14] Ravì, D., Wong, C., Deligianni, F., Berthelot, M., Andreu-Perez, J., Lo, B., and Yang, G.Z., Deep learning for health informatics. *IEEE Journal of Biomedical and Health Informatics,* 21 (1), 4–21, 2016.

[15] Young, T., Hazarika, D., Poria, S., and Cambria, E. Recent trends in deep learning based natural language processing. *IEEE Computational Intelligence Magazine,* 13 (3), 55–75, 2018.

[16] Litjens, G., Kooi, T., Bejnordi, B.E., Setio, A.A.A., Ciompi, F., Ghafoorian, M., Van Der Laak, J.A., Van Ginneken, B., and Sánchez, C.I. A survey on deep learning in medical image analysis. *Medical Image Analysis,* 42, 60–88, 2017.

[17] Schaefer, K. E., Sanders, T. L., Yordon, R. E., Billings, D. R., and Hancock, P. A. Classification of robot form: Factors predicting perceived trustworthiness. In *Proceedings of the Human Factors and Ergonomics Society Annual Meeting,* 56 (1), 1548–1552, Sept. 2012.

[18] Davenport, T. and Kalakota, R. The potential for artificial intelligence in healthcare. *Future Healthcare Journal,* 6 (2), 94, 2019.

[19] Robinson, J. H., Callister, L. C., Berry, J. A., and Dearing, K. A. Patient-centered care and adherence: Definitions and applications to improve outcomes. *Journal of the American Academy of Nurse Practitioners,* 20 (12), 600–607, 2008.

2 Role of Internet of Things and Cloud Computing Technologies in the Healthcare Sector

2.1 INTRODUCTION

A cloud-based healthcare service with the Internet of Healthcare Things (IoHT) is a model to deliver for urbanized regions and vulnerable populations that exploit digital communication. IoHT offers flexible chances to convert health data into workable, personalized health insights, and helps to achieve wellness outside the classical hospital setting. IoT is assumed to be an innovative method with a collection of interlinked objects that link in several cases. IoT methods are capable of having an entire business spectrum because every device is detected with a smart Internet structure, with several advantages. Such merits are comprised of the latest system connections, facilities, and devices that exceed machine-to-machine (M2M) scenarios.

IoT tends to deploy solutions applicable for various domains such as traffic congestion, waste maintenance, smart cities, safety, modern health, logistics, disaster management, healthcare, trade, and business control. Medical, as well as healthcare, show a higher striking application for IoT. IoT is more applicable in improving medical applications such as fitness, primary care, remote health observation, chronic disease management, etc. Compliance with treatment from the home is an alternate significant application. As a result, diverse medical and diagnostic sensors might be tracked concerning smart devices, introducing the required value of the IoT model. Also, it reduces the cost and improves the working function of the model. In previous decades, most of the developers examined IoT's potentials concerning healthcare by assuming diverse real-time applications. Finally, the chapter is comprised of diverse facilities and applications of an area.

IoT is a vital section involved in the research community, public sector, and organizations. Several conventional internets facilitate interaction among devices and humans; IoT links everything with an extensive network of interconnected computing knowledge with no human intervention. The application of IoT and wireless communication approaches enables to monitor the health condition of a patient. Moreover, a greater number of sensors and portable devices are applicable in measuring specific human physiological metrics such as heart rate (HR), respiration rate (RR), and blood pressure (BP).

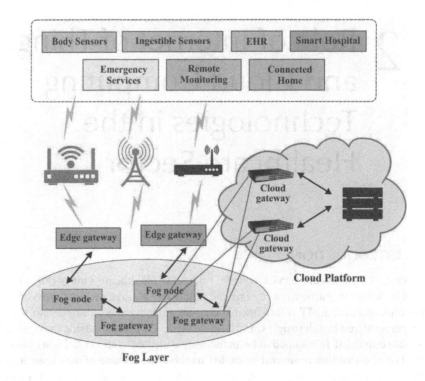

FIGURE 2.1   An overview of a representative IoT and CC-based healthcare scheme.

Although it was present in an earlier phase, businesses and firms have been applied with the energy of IoT, and it is evident that there are improvements in the generation and customer experiences [1]. The combination of IoT in healthcare tends to result in challenging issues, such as data management, information exchange, security as well as privacy, and unified ubiquitous access. A feasible solution that can be used in resolving these issues is present in the CC model. Fig. 2.1 depicts a common healthcare domain that concatenates IoT and CC to offer the capability for using distributed medical data as well as typical structure ubiquitously and transparently, providing on-demand facility, through the system, and meets the challenging problems.

Here, CC provides facilities such as processing of servers, databases, networking, software, and data diagnostics using the Internet, which results in providing rapid installation, reliable resources, and financial scale. Moreover, there has been a recent shift from centralized method CC to the decentralized model (fog computing). Fog computing is utilized to perform data analytics that result in real-time computation, data privacy enhancement, and cost reduction. The increased portable devices, artificial intelligence (AI), and CC assure the organizational base for IoT in healthcare to increase the lifetime of every human. Some of the IoT reviews are experimented by [2] for maximum in-depth as well as highly extensive knowledge regarding maximum factors of IoT to solve maximum problems related to this approach. Therefore, it refers [3] for gaining insights regarding CC and fog computing methodologies, and corresponding applications, different challenges that exist at the time of implementing CC and fog computing, while feasible future works have to be carried out in advance.

IoT offers appropriate solutions for diverse functions that include every aspect of smart cities [4], modern traffic management, waste management, structural health tracking, security, emergency facilities, provide chain, retail, industrial management, and healthcare. Based on a CISCO survey, around 600 billion gadgets will be linked in the future, which is 58 smart devices for every single person. IoT research has been conducted by Statista stating that global IoT studies will attain $8.9 trillion by 2020 from the healthcare sector. Therefore, these merits are accomplished by the combination of IoT and CC in healthcare applications, and health experts providing rapid, effective, as well as optimal healthcare services that tend to be a good user experience. Consequently, it enables to supply optimized healthcare facilities, good patient involvement, and minimized paperwork to health experts.

This chapter performs a survey carried out for analyzing the advanced IoT elements, applications, and market tendency of IoT in healthcare, and the recent growth in IoT and CC-centric healthcare. It also assumes that challenging models such as CC, ambient assisted living, and big data are suitable to apply in healthcare as well as identifying diverse IoT, e-health regulations, and suggestions to compute the way of assisting sustainable growth of IoT as well as CC in the healthcare industry.

2.2 IoT-BASED HEALTHCARE FRAMEWORK

The IoT in healthcare framework (IoTHeF) is assumed to be the basic factor of IoT in healthcare because it provides a complete application of IoT and CC. In addition, it offers supportive messages and transmission of actual medical signals from diverse sensing and modern tools for the fog nodes. As given in Fig. 2.2, it is comprised of three required units of IoTHeF, such as topology, structure, and platform. Every unit is facilitated as particular activities of IoT healthcare application. IoT structures in [5] have been referred to as gaining insights with IoT structures for healthcare. These systems gathered data about patient health conditions by several sensors. Then, the gathered data was forwarded to the remote server to analyze, and the real-time results were displayed.

The IoTHeF architecture defines the arrangement of external IoT units, which is vastly applied among smart devices; a fundamental structure to combine IoT and CC into a modern health solution. Here, a greater number of sensors are applied in

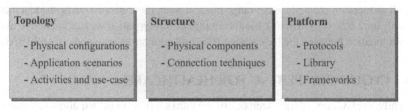

FIGURE 2.2 Three basic modules and their important applications in the IoT framework for healthcare.

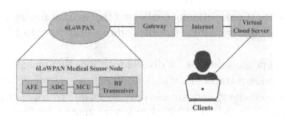

FIGURE 2.3   General IoTHeF design in a medical sensor network.

monitoring patients, collecting data, and the collected data is transferred to a network of sink nodes. Every sink node is identifiable as well as applied by Internet Protocol version 6 (IPv6). Every node is permanent, and sink nodes are more significant by linking with local computers by serial ports. Hence, a gateway-controlled access to the Internet with a border router that performs the action of an IPv6 packet fragmentation management scheme in IPv6 with low-power wireless personal area networks (6LoWPAN).

The sensors are programmed to as sender as well as receiver because it cannot spread by data generated with adjacent nodes. Also, a benchmark Internet engineering task force (IETF) router has been utilized to assure the data collection over multihop by effectively forwarding IPv6 data packets under the application of stable radio connection relied on the IEEE 802.15.4 standard. As a result, to mine a large number of information, a massive information backend server has been developed to assist information gathered as well as hosting. It is employed on CC to save data permanently.

Fig. 2.3 presented by [6] demonstrates a productive IoTHeF infrastructure that emphasizes the gateway; it can be a complete approach of applying analogue tools and 6LoWPAN medical sensors to save bio-signal, contextual, as well as health metrics on CC. The gathered data undergoes investigation on the remote system. At last, the system illustrates the visualized outcome for users. The projected method is comprised with the gateway to transfer health data from diverse sensors to the backend server, a tunneling protocol that assists information transfer among a network 6LoWPAN protocol and network that applies Internet protocol version 4 (IPv4) and IPv6, as well as a socket to examine the patient's health status at present.

Moreover, the gateway has various applications such as local clinical data warehouse, local computation, and a notification scheme to balance maximum information transmission value and enhance robustness. An identical IoTHeF infrastructure is referred to in [7] that is combined with diverse medical devices in remote health monitoring.

Wireless communication methods for IoTHeF are divided into two sets: short-range as well as medium range. In short-range transmission, the transmission is inside a medical body area network (MBAN). Medium-range communication is often applied to assist communication between the base station (BS) and an intermediate node of an MBAN.

2.3   CLOUD COMPUTING FOR HEALTHCARE

Recently, the CC concept has been one of the vital sections in Information Technology (IT). It is comprised of scalability, mobility, and security advantages with offering on-demand CC resources for users. Based on [8], CC is aroused as a supportive of

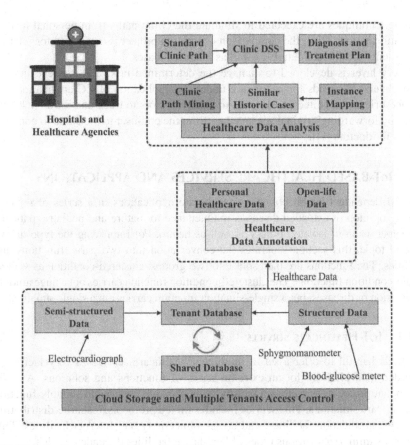

FIGURE 2.4   Functional platform of the CC-dependent m-Health screening scheme.

IoT healthcare applications. An alternate merit of CC is it is capable of sharing data between health experts, caregivers, and patients with highly structured and organized fashion, which reduces the risks of losing medical data. Consequently, healthcare facilities, as well as applications, are acquired from IoT and CC [9]. An environment of an m-Health tracking scheme depends on the CC model that has three major layers presented in [10]; as shown in Fig. 2.4. The Cloud Storage and Multiple Tenants Access Control Layer are assumed to be these applications that obtain healthcare data gathered with sensors like blood pressure (BP) and sphygmomanometers regularly. The cost of saving and managing data has been controlled using the cloud model. Therefore, a greater number of tenant access controls between tenant databases and distributed databases have been executed for improving the security as well as the privacy of patient information. A Healthcare Data Annotation Layer resolves the data heterogeneity problem that often occurs while data processing. The developers presented open Linked Life Data (LLD) groups to annotate healthcare information and combine shared information in a patient-centric design to the CC domain. The Healthcare Data Analysis Layer examines healthcare details saved in CC to help in making clinical decisions the same as with historical data, which are valid assets.

Mining techniques are executed to simulate the clinic paths from personal health-care information. Then, the comparison estimation project is developed for relating the patients' healthcare details as well as historical cases.

Every layer is developed to manage the determined task, and it is executed to serve diverse demands for healthcare under the application of CC application and service-oriented architecture. It tends to enable doctors to track and estimate health status by forwarding original sensors data from the end-user to the cloud to compute results for doctors [11].

2.4 IoT-BASED HEALTHCARE SERVICES AND APPLICATIONS

The IoT-dependent health observing results are applications in a series of regions, namely opinion of extended diseases, maintenance to mature and pediatric patients, and supervision of isolated fitness as well as health. For improving the type of this general topic, this section separates the conversation into two parts: functions and facilities. The functions are then split into two groups: clustered-condition as well as single-condition functions. The clustered-condition function carries out a huge amount of situation or diseases, but a single-situation function carries out a single situation.

2.4.1 IoT Healthcare Services

IoT finds helpful to offer a set of intelligent healthcare services. Every facility is regarded as a platform for an extreme series of functions and solutions. An IoT-dependent protocol, as well as a facility's, needs small changes to suitably function in healthcare situations. This service includes linked protocols, resource-distributing facilities, notification facilities, and cross-connectivity and Internet facilities. This segment summarizes various types of healthcare facilities dependent on IoT.

2.4.1.1 The Internet of m-Health Things

M-health is a group of medical sensing, mobile, as well as transmission skills to healthcare services. It observes execution problems, Internet of m-health Things (m-IoT) structure, and tasks of noninvasive glucose level sensing.

2.4.1.2 Adverse Drug Reactions

The adverse drug response denotes harmful or unpleasant reaction resulting from an intervention relevant to the utilization of a medicinal product.

2.4.1.3 Community Healthcare

Community healthcare indicates the formation of a network that is a part of public health that concentrates on people and their responsibilities as determinants of their own and other people's health [12].

2.4.1.4 Children's Health Information

Increasing attention and enhancing education regarding children through mental as well as sensitive issues and to require among the common public and their family members is important.

2.4.2 IoT HEALTHCARE APPLICATIONS

Additionally, IoT facility's or IoT healthcare functions need closer attention. It can be taken into account that functions need facilities before they are utilized with patients. So, functions are developed as user-centric. In this subsection, the various functions of healthcare that depend on IoT, including both clustered as well as unique functions, are explained.

2.4.2.1 Glucose Level Sensing

Diabetes is a metabolic disease that raises the glucose level. Observing glucose represents changes in blood forms and actions. An actual glucose level observing method was established.

2.4.2.2 Electrocardiogram Monitoring

The electrocardiogram (ECG) displays the electrical measure of a human heart, defining the beat as well as HR, QT intervals, myocardial ischemia, and analysis of arrhythmias. Yang et al. [13] studied IoT-dependent results in ECG screening.

2.4.2.3 Blood Pressure Monitoring

Puustjärvi and Puustjärvi [14] utilized the instance of BP observing as well as a regulator in developing countries as the situation in that telemedicine is an appreciated device.

2.4.2.4 Body Temperature Monitoring

Observing body temperature is a dynamic quantity of medical facilities because it regards a dynamic suggestion of protection of homeostasis. Istepanian et al. [15] confirmed the m-IoT approach utilizing body temperature sensing detected in TelosB motes.

2.4.3 IoT HEALTHCARE: CURRENT ISSUES AND CHALLENGES

Different researchers showed attention to the executing and scheming of various IoT healthcare structures and resolving several building difficulties connected to individual structures. But there are still problems as well as tasks that need to be correctly reported.

2.4.3.1 Cost Analysis

Analysts need the formation of minimum-cost models of IoT-allowed medication results; but, to date, no researchers have regarded this issue.

2.4.3.2 Continuous Monitoring

In a few situations, enduring patient health observing is needed. For accomplishing this, nonstop logging and observing are important.

2.4.3.3 Identification

Healthcare associations and hospitals frequently carry a massive number of patients. For obtaining suitable information management in these conditions, the correct recognition of patients, as well as staff, is vital.

2.4.3.4 Mobility

IoT healthcare solutions are accomplished in supporting the flexibility of patients as they are connected whenever, anyplace. A mobility description is utilized to attach various patients to several networks.

2.5 COMPONENTS IN IoT-BASED HEALTHCARE SERVICES

2.5.1 IoT Devices

IoT tools are little in size, function on a minimum power source, and have restricted processing size. Microcontrollers through 8-bit as well as 16-bit processors are well-identified in the market. The focused foreground-background technique is utilized to a single processor for managing multiple procedures at a time. The processors with an 8-bit or 16-bit manner are not particular to planarity for supporting IoT tools, and this tool uses a present operating system (OS). The actual OS needs further energy as well as memory and higher developing abilities to be employed through tools.

There are also several other problems for tools to work in the IoT paradigm. If a device can assist Transmission Control Protocol/Internet Protocol (TCP/IP) stack to network, then this stack is not an easy program, because additional random-access memory (RAM) is essential to manage the count of network buffers to TCP. Also, Java assist is appealing to an IoT tool; so, Java Virtual Machine (JVM) must be functioning on the OS of IoT tools. In the end, RAM and read-only memory (ROM) assist must be feasible to IoT tools for supporting the actual OS and transmission stack. Nowadays, a 32-bit microcontroller unit that is tiny in size, functions on the minimum power source, and has enough processing size for supporting IoT tools are also accessible on the market. These 32-bit microcontroller units are the optimal choice for IoT creators as well as providers.

Data acquisition, firmware upgrade, power management, communication stack, processing, protocol alteration, and customizable security features are executed in IoT tools with utilizing 32-bit microcontroller units. An Intel and ARM family is well-identified in the market of 32-bit structure processors. The Intel family gives assistance to industrial Internet functions through atom processors, as the Intel Quark also apprehensions the embedded scheme market. Instead, the ARM Cortex-M0 processor is particular to give a minimum-cost product to IoT methods. ARM Cortex-M3, M4, and M7 are the optimal opinions for creating IoT gateway tools. Higher action, energy stability, and suitable scheme edges are the main attributes of these processors to support IoT gateways.

For supporting minimum energy utilization and higher action, the RL78 is the better 16-bit processor in the novel creation of Renesas microcontrollers. Several opponents to microcontroller units are giving their market resolutions by pros and cons, then assisting smart and little-embedded schemes, ARM, Intel, and Renesas are famous and well verified. For assisting little IoT resource-controlled tools, Oracle's Java ME embedded has been planned. Java ME Embedded 8 is extremely utilized in wireless components, buildings, industrial manages, health schemes, grid observing, and several further functions. The Java ME Embedded 8 needs the schemes depending on the ARM structure system-on-chips (SOCs) to have 128 KB of RAM, and

1 MB of ROM, contain an easy embed kernel or OS, and have a network link that is also wired or wireless. The Java ME Embedded 8 is also between the minimum-cost results and appropriate for supporting resource-particular tools of an IoT method.

2.5.2 WIRELESS TECHNOLOGIES FOR IoT

Usual communication technologies are needed for an IoT method. To communicate among IoT tools as well as backend facility providers, the communication technology must be selected. An IoT tool is allowed through wireless attachment. Without single ordinary wireless technology for supporting an IoT model, the amount of technology that contains pros, as well as cons, are accessible. Execution of wireless technology is also based on the IoT scheme. For instance, a healthcare scheme or an environment-observing scheme. The connection between a few wireless technologies is provided.

2.5.3 WEB TECHNOLOGIES FOR IoT

Present web progress is utilized for IoT methods. But this process is not enough to correctly assist IoT methods; so, outcomes are worse. JSON, as well as XML, is distributed in payloads with utilizing HTTP and WebSocket protocols. Predefined web protocols are executed on IoT tools, then this protocol needs further reserves for supporting IoT functions. For supporting IoT methods, several particular protocols have been established that work effectively through reserve-controlled IoT tools and networks.

2.6 CONCLUSION

This chapter has shown how to analyze up-to-date IoT modules, functions, and market movements of IoT in healthcare, and learning present progress in IoT and CC-based healthcare functions. It regards how capable technologies, namely CC, ambient supported living, big data, as well as wearables, are presently executed in the healthcare trade and finds different IoT, e-health rules, and procedures worldwide that support the maintainable progress of IoT as well as CC in the healthcare trade. This chapter has provided details about IoT and cloud technologies for the healthcare environment.

REFERENCES

[1] Asif-Ur-Rahman, M., Afsana, F., Mahmud, M., Kaiser, M.S., Ahmed, M.R., Kaiwartya, O. and James-Taylor, A. Toward a heterogeneous mist, fog, and cloud-based framework for the internet of healthcare things. *IEEE Internet of Things Journal*, 6 (3), 4049–4062, 2018.

[2] Lakshmanaprabu, S. K., Mohanty, S. N., Krishnamoorthy, S., Uthayakumar, J., and Shankar, K. Online clinical decision support system using optimal deep neural networks. *Applied Soft Computing*, 81, 105487, 2019.

[3] Shankar, K., Lakshmanaprabu, S. K., Gupta, D., Maseleno, A., and De Albuquerque, V. H. C. Optimal feature-based multi-kernel SVM approach for thyroid disease classification. *The Journal of Supercomputing*, 1–16, 2018.

[4] Lakshmanaprabu, S. K., Mohanty, S. N., Shankar, K., Arunkumar, N., and Ramirez, G. Optimal deep learning model for classification of lung cancer on CT images. *Future Generation Computer Systems*, 92, 374–382, 2019.

[5] Shankar, K., Elhoseny, M., Lakshmanaprabu, S. K., Ilayaraja, M., Vidhyavathi, R. M., Elsoud, M. A., and Alkhambashi, M. Optimal feature level fusion based ANFIS classifier for brain MRI image classification. *Concurrency and Computation: Practice and Experience*, e4887, 1–12, 2018.

[6] Gia, T.N., Thanigaivelan, N.K., Rahmani, A.M., Westerlund, T., Liljeberg, P., and Tenhunen, H. Customizing 6LoWPAN networks towards Internet-of-Things based ubiquitous healthcare systems. In Proceedings of the 2014 NORCHIP, Tampere, Finland, October 27–28, 2014, 1–6.

[7] Elhoseny, M., Bian, G. B., Lakshmanaprabu, S. K., Shankar, K., Singh, A. K., and Wu, W. Effective features to classify ovarian cancer data in internet of medical things. *Computer Networks*, 159, 147–156, 2019.

[8] Sultan, N. Making use of cloud computing for healthcare provision: Opportunities and, challenges. *International Journal of Information Management,* 34, 177–184, 2014.

[9] Darwish, A., Hassanien, A.E., Elhoseny, M., Sangaiah, A.K., and Muhammad, K. The impact of the hybrid platform of Internet of Things and cloud computing on healthcare systems: Opportunities, challenges, and open problems. *Journal of Ambient Intelligence and Humanized Computing*, 10, 1–16, 2017.

[10] Xu, B., Xu, L., Cai, H., Jiang, L., Luo, Y., and Gu, Y. The design of an m-Health monitoring system based on a cloud computing platform. *Enterprise Information Systems*, 11, 17–36, 2017.

[11] Singh, D., Tripathi, G., Alberti, A.M., and Jara, A. Semantic edge computing and IoT architecture for military health services in battlefield. In Proceedings of the 2017 14th IEEE Annual Consumer Communications & Networking Conference (CCNC), Las Vegas, Nevada, USA, January 8–11, 2017, 185–190.

[12] Rohokale, V. M., Prasad, N. R, and Prasad, R. A cooperative Internet of Things (IoT) for rural healthcare monitoring and control. In 2nd International Conference on Wireless Communication, Vehicular Technology, Information Theory and Aerospace & Electronic Systems Technology (Wireless VITAE). IEEE, 2011.

[13] Yang, G., et al. A health-IoT platform based on the integration of intelligent packaging, unobtrusive bio-sensor, and intelligent medicine box. *IEEE Transactions on Industrial Informatics*, 10 (4), 2180–2191, 2014.

[14] Puustjärvi, J., and Puustjärvi, L. Automating remote monitoring and information therapy: An opportunity to practice telemedicine in developing countries. In IST-Africa Conference Proceedings, IEEE, 2011.

[15] Istepanian, R. S., et al. The potential of Internet of m-Health Things "m-IoT" for noninvasive glucose level sensing. In Engineering in Medicine and Biology Society, EMBC, Annual International Conference of the IEEE, 2011.

3 An Extensive Overview of Wearable Technologies in the Healthcare Sector

3.1 INTRODUCTION

In recent times, the Internet of Health Things (IoHT) has become more popular in the healthcare sector, which generally includes a collection of the interlinked infrastructure of medicinal gadgets, software applications, and health systems and services. The utilization of the Internet of Things (IoT) in the medicinal field has abruptly raised several IoT use cases in the industry, personal healthcare, and healthcare payment applications. Wearable technology (WT) encloses the plethora of devices that are fixed with a transient connection. The secondary method contains smart mobiles, which are referred to as a core part of WT function. Although it is composed with the definition of smartphones as WT, the presence of the demise and rebirth of WT becomes more applicable in routine lifestyle [1]. This is due to the increase of cybercrime, a high cost of well-equipped applications. Also, mobile computation is highly influential, which is one of the significant innovations in WT such as processing rapid, robust, and simple bioassays at any place and time. WT is further divided into two classes: primary and secondary. The initial stage of primary deals with the independent operation in central connectors of alternate data, for instance, wrist-worn fitness trackers and smartphones, while the secondary class contributes to capturing particular events such as heart rate monitoring [2]. These classes are also included with modern textiles in which external features of the material can estimate stimuli from a user.

Some of the modern textiles leading to improving the value of the daily application of wearing digital tailored materials inside clothes or directly on skin retains the vernacular of scientific researchers. Regardless, fueled by miniaturization of electronic-based units, WT experiences the evolution of the primary condition to acquire conventional desktop computing. The WT has the capability of collecting and recording data and processing tedious computations, in healthcare applications, WT is realized as applicable devices to examine the patient status, remedy, as well as controlling of the disease. Regulatory bodies, as well as vendors providing medical applications, struggle for distinguishing apps as clinical tools that require normal regulatory acceptance, versus the well-trained user market. Fig. 3.1 shows the structure of wearables in healthcare applications.

The quality of a device and the application of diverse standards to analyze the accuracy with standard rate and interaction interoperability are interwoven by

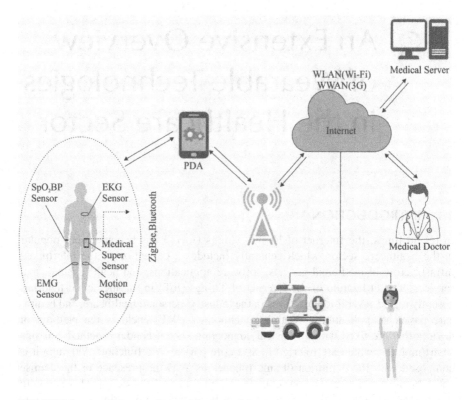

FIGURE 3.1 Architecture of wearables in healthcare.

projecting additional obstacles for medical consumption of WT. The purpose of this application is to review and highlight the important factors of WTs at minimum effective application for healthcare. Recently, it has been applied with a myriad of methodologies that have lower popularity in this domain.

WT has various electronic-centric sensors based on required values such as electrocardiogram (ECG) and blood glucose. These sensors produce an electrical signal while predicting physiological symptoms, which is captured several times for measurement demand. Consecutively, signals are recorded as difficult time series data by the data electronics. Off-the-shelf commercial tools apply proprietary software with integrated methods for downloading data, obtaining required information features, and producing essential results. Also, several WTs provides permission to use the actual data for developing bespoke methodologies through research gadgets such as MATLAB® for maximum insightful patient estimation. Consequently, it decides on the open-source developing choice in deploying techniques when compared with black box models.

The technologies were shaped based on computer-relied protocols for computing the sections of original electronic signals to obtain real-time information, the reliable outcome. It is considered to be more tedious from the permutations of data interpretation; however, pseudocode presentations give few insights for the task such as eye tracking [3]. WT is capable of frequently monitoring several iterations. Therefore, it has negative battery replacement as well as storage abilities and improved data capturing minimized WT installation duration. Although WT could apply maximum batteries, it makes WT ineffective by being too large to wear discretely. While applying WT, data acquisition is essential for ensuring data gathering strategies. For instance, minimum data and possible clues for analyzing patient details might be imputed; later, the searching process in big data in the case of clinically sensitive results is more tedious.

Generally, it is placed in low-power mode and speeds up the extra sensors if there is a feasible action that can be predicted. Big data is gathered in a free-living atmosphere that provides habitual nature such as seasonal movements and absence of direct medicinal observation. The major barrier that is present in applying big data inside a healthcare domain is selecting the best structure for memory, such as Structured Query Language (SQL) and analytical methods such as Apache Hive, which is not suitable [4].

Several WTs become a portion of IoT: connecting to electronic communication structures, serving fast data exchange as well as storage. The IoT devices generates a gigabytes (GB) of data for regular application. It is mainly based on the impact of hardware deployment on capturing the physiological values.

Following that, stable WT is optimally served as supervised patient estimation while instrumented testing in generic platforms with high sensitive electronic-based data. WT provides habitual information of serving self-care, a WT link with cloud computing (CC), adheres to GDPR, and guarantees ubiquitous sensing abilities in which embedded machine learning (ML) or artificial intelligence (AI) systems decipher from big data. Finally, WT data on a cloud is used by healthcare experts from a search engine, which makes the process simpler for users.

Feedback from these health services has to be employed in developing tasks. The cusp of the yottabyte (YB) period requires the size of big data that can be used as large proportions. The cloud is capable of resolving the constraints by offering a ubiquitous computerized financial scale: the energy of an effective system can be employed anywhere by different devices. However, CC is a developed optimizing technique, such as fogs and cloudlets for processing data present in network edges. Therefore, the study involved in this approach is named edge computing while realistic analysis is more important to increase the data efficiency [5].

3.2 BACKGROUND INFORMATION

Massive terms are used in defining monitored health data, such as "quantified self" and "WT." The known differences of these models will be useful in medical practice as well as patient results.

3.2.1 QUANTIFIED SELF

The quantified self migrations are initialized as an attempt to define the application of personal fitness trackers by *WIRED* magazine writers Gary Wolf and Kevin Kelly, while the method is comprised of a novel new culture of observing and distributing personal data. It is the major portion of monitoring data with the application of smartphones and wearables such as smartwatches as well as Fitbits. WT automatic data collection applies the methodologies for examining data and provides repeated data. Wearables are embraced by people because the automatic journal does not depend upon user access and data; rather, it frequently tracks the user device. Hence, it is named as quantified selfers using the personal mathematical data gathered from wearables for events like eating, sleeping, exercising, and regular habits. Quantified selfers believe that it enhances the factors of regular lifestyle.

3.2.2   WEARABLE TECHNOLOGY

Fitness trackers are said to be simple wearables and observe a massive amount of personal data, such as steps, heart rate, power cost, sleep patterns, and so on. An alternate type of wearable are smart glasses, which are an optical head-coated display modeled in the form of eyeglasses. Additionally, smart-wearable devices are observing the functions of the human heart; contact lenses observe glucose levels and eye pressure; headbands help in capturing electroencephalograms; camera technology is applied in examining outer values of mental health by composite data, namely, tone, inflection, as well as facial expressions; and shirts are embedded with the method to estimate cardiac metrics.

Recently, smartwatches exploded onto the market. They are unobtrusive and fit lifestyles as well as perform fundamental tracking while paired with smartphones. Eric Topol, physician and futurist, believes smartphones are capable of reducing the workload of doctors, cutting expenses, improving the practice of care, and providing maximum energy for patients [6]. Recent work under the application of smartwatches aims at chronic populations; although there is more research on wearables on depression, Parkinson's disease, and heart disease (HD) [7]. Fig. 3.2 depicts the user wearable model.

3.2.3   ADVANTAGES OF WEARABLE TECHNOLOGY

Healthcare is highly applied by patients in remote sites. Patients do not move, but rather forward the data with transient visits with nurse practitioners (NPs). Lay caregivers could obtain the merits of applying data from wearables for observing aged patients and alternate homebound patients. Wearables could offer data like steps, sleeping patterns, and ECG, with automated examination. Such data helps NPs diagnose problems and intervene rapidly for preventing readmissions, since it is comprised of high insight in regular patient functions. Also, wearables collect data in an automated manner to resolve restricted memory storage. This helps NPs to have an extensive view of a patient. With the application of pedometers, physical activity can be improved and reduce blood pressure (BP) as well as body mass index (BMI).

3.3   CHALLENGES

The problems involved might balance out the merits. Even though the benefits of wearables are high, there are problems involved to solve such as an improved application by NPs, as well as patient's data.

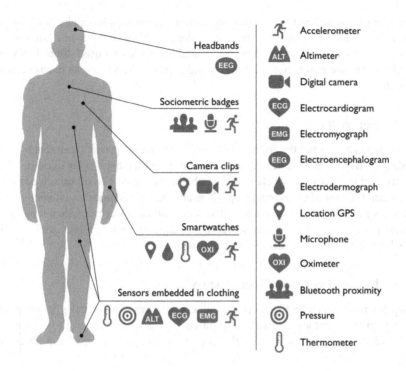

FIGURE 3.2 Consumer wearable.

3.3.1 SUSTAINABILITY

Shankar et al. [8] presented a method of frequent employment of devices in four levels:

- Level 1 is an original decision for monitoring data under the application of a wearable. Usually, it tracks data for a particular reason such as weight loss or to boost health, and applies devices to perform a task.
- Level 2 selects the desired device, used in selecting cost and features, and also the value of user trust in attaining the goal.
- Level 3 combines with data observed, understands data, and makes useful as well as positive modifications.
- Level 4 is lapsing, which terminates self-monitoring with the probability of repeating the application. For some reason, users stop using the wearable, such as cost, technique failure, absence of interest, and so on. Since wearables are convenient and effective, retained employment would improve outcomes.

3.3.2 DIGITAL DIVIDE

The application of WT has increased with millennials. Users facing challenging issues, such as minimum profit, rural, and homebound populations, merit from wearables. The International Telecommunication Union, the United Nations' official source for global data as well as communications techniques, has addressed that low income households also have online access along with the high income households. With no access to the Internet at home, wearables cannot be used often. It divides the NPs as an essential factor for patients and expands the variations in case among populations.

3.3.3 FAILURE RATES

The medical gadgets has the ability to examine and provide proper treatment by turning the mobile screen for a device. They can be supported by varying data, stability, validity, and accuracy. Every class of wearable device results in minimum accuracy to evaluate the cost of measuring steps. The absence of accuracy and device failure of devices provides a conundrum for NPs. When data is not correct, then it has to be applied in direct care. Patients do not learn the requirement for validity, and stability of such devices believes in data as they are factual.

3.3.4 LACK OF PREDICTIVE COMPARABILITY

Generally, research cannot support the evidence that wearables make people stronger. Applying wearables is healthier when compared with a user who is not monitored. Additionally, it is addressed that a certain number of people stop observing data around a year.

3.3.5 PRIVACY AND SECURITY

Agreement for devices' terms and conditions belongs to the employment of data. While processing the consent task, users allow the researcher to distribute data from third parties to market the research process. There are certain methods of tracking that appear intrusive, and patients might be resistant to utilize the data. In [9], while provided with a tracking model of blood glucose with type II diabetes, patients exhibited maximum values on the depression subscale while using self-trackers. Also, patients became over-reliant on observed data and ineffective self-diagnosis.

Based on the seven-country report, 7,000 healthcare customers, and NPs, wish to apply the observed data, but clear parameters are essential. Even though NPs are willing to employ patient-produced data, combining data with a patient's Electronic Health Record (EHR) cannot be simply achieved.

3.4 TYPICAL WEARABLE DEVICES WITH APPLICATIONS IN HEALTH

Wearables that are often applied to medical sectors enclose biochemical sensors. Biochemical sensors are vastly applied in computing glucose, alcohol, electrolyte, pH, oxygenation, and gas, humidity. They are combined with a chemically sensible layer and a transducer to transform a chemical analyte into an electrical signal. They are also applied for calculating internal and external chemicals as well as biochemical species in health tracking.

3.4.1 WEARABLE DEVICES USED FOR GENERAL HEALTH MANAGEMENT

Wearable devices offer the chance to enhance healthcare in diverse settings, from in-hospital care, for ambulance care in the home and remote sites, as well as in rural areas and low-resource platforms. The main problem of the wider application in healthcare is obtaining applicable data and useful health-based data from a massive amount of data. This has emerged from anticipated developing scope and the healthcare landscape worldwide by giving options in the automated prediction of health actions and installation of movable interventions.

Data analyzing models such as ML exhibit a promising objective to extend the application of wearables into medical sectors, which range from detecting acute health actions to observing chronic diseases like HD and diabetes. Here, the consumption of wearable sensors is controlling health and disease diagnosis; participants wear devices such as user fitness trackers. Such tools measure the external events, heart rate, skin as well as ambient temperature, electrodermal activity, blood oxygen saturation, and radiation exposure [10].

In addition, the performance of clinical and biomolecular values like multi-omics as a portion of the Integrative Personal Omics Profiling study takes place. It is easy to detect the medical rates of inflammation, infection, and insulin sensitivity conditions based on values of a user's smartwatch [11]. The application of people fitness trackers and personalized creations are used in tracking a user's health status. PhysIQ is a major instance of detecting subtle modifications of a patient's baseline with the help of bio-sensing tools for offering real-world health issues [12].

3.4.2 WEARABLE BIOSENSORS REVOLUTIONIZING IN-CLINIC/HOSPITAL CARE

Historical tools are used in collecting patient details from a clinic or emergency department (ED), which serves as faster triaging to offer adverse care for patients with more demand. Developers receive optimal feedback on perceived applicability in wearing trackables in ED settings from patients and caretakers [13]. Recently, it has been identified with the application of important symbols in automatic triage of ED patients. Levin et al. [14] implied an ML-relied system named e-triage that applies input patient significant signs, chief complaint, and active medical data. In a multisite retrospective ED visit, e-triage detections receive the characteristic curve of 0.73 to 0.92. E-triage is executed at Johns Hopkins Medicine to validate research works.

Moreno et al. [15] expanded the model by deploying bracelets for patients in ED; although, it is not sampled for calculating the efficiency of patient triage. In hospital inpatient care, constant observation is applied in multiparameter patient signs like BP, blood oxygen saturation [SpO2], heart rate, and respiration rate. However, patients are comprised of complications as they move to several hospitals with more tracking devices. A wireless nature of novel wearable sensors that calculate the predefined possible signs and extra metrics such as movement, skin conductance, food, self-care and bathroom habits, and so on, improves patient tracking in hospital settings at the time of enhancing patient comfort as well as mobility [16].

3.4.3 WEARABLE BIOSENSORS REVOLUTIONIZING SPECIFIC FIELDS OF HEALTHCARE OUTSIDE OF THE HOSPITAL AND CLINIC

Wearable sensors are used in diverse healthcare-based applications, such as common well-being, extensive medical care, condition-based monitoring, as well as mobile health deployments. This has been defined with the wearables employed in the outside world for metabolic, cardiovascular, and gastrointestinal observation; neurology and mental health; maternal, prenatal, and neonatal care; as well as pulmonary health and ecological exposures.

3.4.4 REGULATORY OVERSIGHT AND ECONOMIC IMPACT

The US Food and Drug Administration (FDA) monitor electronic health classes such as mobile health (mHealth), health data technique, WT, telehealth and telemedicine, and personalized medicine. The FDA published a digital health software pilot program to concentrate on developing software models, verification, and provision by electronic health-based organizations.

The nine companies chosen to participate were Apple (CA, USA), Fitbit, Johnson & Johnson (CA, USA), Pear Therapeutics (CA, USA), Phosphorous (NY, USA), Roche (CA, USA), Samsung (SKR), Tidepool (CA, USA), and Verily. Wireless medical tools are combined by the Federal Communications Commission and the FDA is employed to regularize the convergence of medical tools with connections as well as useful methods by Centers for Medicare and Medicaid Services (CMS) to estimate the expense of market regulation [17]. A dense database through the FDA is called the Recognized Consensus Standards database. Several devices are defined in Wireless Medical Telemetry Systems. The FDA explains wireless medical telemetry as a system that is often employed in monitoring patient's vital symptoms such as pulse and respiration with the help of radio frequency communication, which has the merits of enabling patient actions without any limitations to track with hardware connection. A massive number of tools have recently been used by the FDA, which is capable of changing the healthcare landscape as provided with the exploitation of clinic disease control. By interchanging five outpatient consultations and home visits, it can save the maximum amount over a year of hospital expenses [17]. In this study, a total of 43 patient data with is gathered using implantable cardiovascular gadgets ($n = 43$), and remote healthcare monitoring is provided with reduced cost. It also reduces the overhead of the hospital.

3.5 CONCLUSION

The disruptive behavior of WT tends to slow deployment in today's healthcare. The potential of WT as a pragmatic and clinically applicable method to aid patient diagnosis, treatment, and care is more evident. This is because of the low-cost ability to collect habitual information from a discrete manner for longitudinal periods at any platform. A combination of cloud offers accessible big data, serving the domain of ML approaches in new simulation outcomes. Therefore, limited data management and proper validation procedures are absent in the approach with predetermined learning processes. Regardless, WT is rife and still an R&D phase of the life cycle. The parallel execution of exact data regulation, validation models, ubiquitous concatenation to global networks, and improved generations would see WT realizing process.

REFERENCES

[1] Kathiresan, S., Sait, A. R. W., Gupta, D., Lakshmanaprabu, S. K., Khanna, A., and Pandey, H. M. Automated detection and classification of fundus diabetic retinopathy images using synergic deep learning model. *Pattern Recognition Letters*, 133, 210–216, 2020.

[2] Cadmus-Bertram L. Using fitness trackers in clinical research: what nurse practitioners need to know. *Journal for Nurse Practitioners*, 13 (1), 34–40, 2017.

[3] Shankar, K., Perumal, E., and Vidhyavathi, R. M. Deep neural network with moth search optimization algorithm based detection and classification of diabetic retinopathy images. *SN Applied Sciences*, 2(4), 1–10, 2020.

[4] S. Sakr, and Elgammal, A. Towards a comprehensive data analytics framework for smart healthcare services, *Big Data Research*, 4, 44–58, 2016.

[5] Asif-Ur-Rahman, M., Afsana, F., Mahmud, M., Kaiser, M.S., Ahmed, M.R., Kaiwartya, O. and James-Taylor, A., Toward a heterogeneous mist, fog, and cloud-based framework for the internet of healthcare things. *IEEE Internet of Things Journal*, 6 (3), 4049–4062, 2018.

[6] Elhoseny, M., Shankar, K., and Uthayakumar, J. Intelligent Diagnostic Prediction and Classification System for Chronic Kidney Disease. *Scientific Reports*, 9 (1), 1–14, 2019.

[7] Elhoseny, M., and Shankar, K. Optimal bilateral filter and convolutional neural network based denoising method of medical image measurements. *Measurement*, 143, 125–135, 2019.

[8] Shankar, K., Lakshmanaprabu, S. K., Khanna, A., Tanwar, S., Rodrigues, J. J., and Roy, N. R. Alzheimer detection using Group Grey Wolf Optimization based features with convolutional classifier. *Computers & Electrical Engineering*, 77, 230–243, 2019.

[9] Ruckenstein, M., and Pantzar, M. Beyond the quantified self: thematic exploration of a dataistic paradigm. *New Media & Society*, 19 (3), 401–418, 2017. https://doi.org/10.1177/1461444815609081.

[10] Ballinger B., Hsieh J., and Singh A., et al. DeepHeart: semi-supervised sequence learning for cardiovascular risk prediction. *arXiv*, 2018. https://arxiv.org/abs/1802.02511

[11] Li X., Dunn J., and Salins D., et al. Digital health: tracking physiomes and activity using wearable biosensors reveals useful health-related information. *PLoS Biology*, 15 (1), e2001402, 2017.

[12] Steinhubl S. R., Feye D., Levine A. C., Conkright C., Wegerich S. W., and Conkright G. Validation of a portable, deployable system for continuous vital sign monitoring using a multiparametric wearable sensor and personalised analytics in an Ebola treatment centre. *BMJ Global Health*, 1 (1), e000070, 2016.

[13] Claudio D, Velazquez M. A., Bravo-Llerena W., Okudan G. E., and Freivalds A. Perceived usefulness and ease of use of wearable sensor-based systems in emergency departments. *IIE Transactions on Occupational Ergonomics and Human Factors,* 3 (3–4), 177–187, 2015.

[14] Levin, S., Toerper, M., Hamrock, E., Hinson, J.S., Barnes, S., Gardner, H., Dugas, A., Linton, B., Kirsch, T. and Kelen, G. Machine-learning-based electronic triage more accurately differentiates patients with respect to clinical outcomes compared with the emergency severity index. *Annals of emergency medicine*, 71(5), 565–574, 2018.

[15] Moreno S., Quintero A., Ochoa C., Bonfante M., Villareal R., and Pestana J. Remote monitoring system of vital signs for triage and detection of anomalous patient states in the emergency room. In 2016 XXI Symposium on Signal Processing, Images and Artificial Vision (STSIVA). Bucaramanga, Colombia, August 30–September 2, 2016.

[16] Kroll R. R., McKenzie E. D., and Boyd J. G., et al. Use of wearable devices for post-discharge monitoring of ICU patients: a feasibility study. *Journal of Intensive Care* 5, 64, 2017.

[17] US Food and Drug Administration/Center for Devices and Radiological Health. Wireless medical devices. 2018. www.fda.gov/MedicalDevices/def ault.htm

[18] Atluri V., Cordina J., Mango P., and Velamooret S. How tech-enabled consumers are reordering the healthcare landscape. McKinsey & Company, 2016. www.mckinsey.com/industries/healthcare-systems-and-services/our-insights/how-tech-enabled-consumers-are-reordering-the-healthcare-landscape

4 IoHT and Cloud-Based Disease Diagnosis Model Using Particle Swarm Optimization with Artificial Neural Networks

4.1 INTRODUCTION

In general, Internet of Things (IoT) is defined as the process of developing Internet-linked Things over computer systems. IoT states that rather having low power processing devices such as laptops, tablets, and smartphones, it is optimal to have a minimum number of effective gadgets such as wristbands, air conditioners, umbrellas, and refrigerators. Constant human applicable things such as air fresheners and transport has been smartly deployed using processing units, guided by sensors, and produces practical results, which are incorporated in regular devices. Therefore, the linked things are composed of processing as well as communicating abilities by applying tools such as the average lamp or umbrella to link with network communication. The improved objects in IoT have technical reasoning to process the declared operation with no details of a name and feature or character. The domains of technical expertise and electronics have integrated IoHT, an important scientific advancement. IoHT has started to be used in diverse areas.

The term "ubiquitous computing" varies but generally means computing that is available anytime, anywhere and can be processed over a wide range of Internet. The term "Thing" or object represents that the real world is capable of receiving inputs from humans and converts the obtained data to the Internet to process data gathering. For instance, a sewing machine is capable of recording a thread, values of stitches sewn, and the number of stitches the machine can perform. It is more feasible under the application of sensors while recording the function presented by an object with a limited time interval. Actuators could be employed in a sensor node to show the simulation outcome to the real world by linking the objects. These results are enabled by data collected and deal with the Internet.

IoT and cloud computing (CC) have more advantageous features with equal intensity while combining IoT and CC models. The observing method is deployed by integrating two methodologies to track the patient's data in an effective manner even in remote areas, which is more useful for medical practitioners. IoT schemes often support CC to improvise the function with respect to maximum resource consumption, memory, power, as well as processing ability. Furthermore, CC gains merits from IoT by the improvement of handling the present world and delivers a massive number of novel services in dynamic as well as shared fashion. An IoT-centric CC approach would be expanded for designing fresh methods in the modern world. The concatenation of CC and IoT relying on web fields operates quite well when compared with traditional CC-based domains by means of efficiency.

There are a few novel applications such as the medical, armed forces, and banking sectors that apply the integration of IoT and CC. These combinations would be applicable to provide effective services in medical applications to observe the data from remote sites. IoT-based healthcare domains are employed for collecting required information such as dynamic modifications in health metrics and extend the intensity of medical parameters at the standard time interval. Additionally, IoT tools, as well as medical parameters-based sensor values, are employed effectively to diagnose the disease at the right time prior to attaining a serious condition. As an inclusion, machine learning (ML) techniques are one of the important modules in the decision-making process in the case of large-scale data. The function of applying data analysis for particular regions contributes to data types such as velocity, variety, and volume. The reputed data analysis encloses a neural network (NN), a classification approach, as well as a clustering technique and efficient methodologies.

Data can be produced from diverse sources with specific data types that are more vital in deploying models for handling data features. For IoT, numerous amounts of resources practically develop the required data with no issues of scalability and velocity to find the optimal data method. These factors are assumed to be significant problems of IoT. Here, it is gathered with a large amount of big data that has diverse data such as image, text, and classifying data by applying IoT devices as input data. Such data would be saved in the CC platform with secured healthcare applications. This is employed with a novel ML approach to process the learning function that maps data into two classes: "Normal" and "Disease Affected."

Diverse works have been carried out by several studies over the last few decades [1]. Verma and Sood [2] established a novel approach to monitor the disease intensity and analyzed under the application of CC and IoT. This is mainly applied for detecting the severity of the disease. The core terms are extended for producing user-relied health values that identify a processing science model. Also, it is employed to observe student health data. In this method, a programmatic health data in student point is produced with the application of a reputed UCI Repository and sensors applied in the medicinal sector to forecast diverse diseases that are affected with severity. It is employed with different classifying techniques to detect diverse diseases. The prediction accuracy is calculated for this model by applying metrics such as F-measure, specificity, and sensitivity. Consequently, it is evident that this method performs better with respect to prediction accuracy when compared to conventional approaches.

Li et al. [3] projected novel energy schemes that operate in end-to-end for CC-based IoT platforms. The energy frameworks are used in examining video stream that is generated by vehicles cameras. It is estimated on the basis of practical testbeds, in particular applications that perform the operations with the application of popular simulators to learn the improvement of IoT devices. Stergiou et al. [4] deployed a review on CC and IoT methods with security problems. Furthermore, it is listed with the contribution of CC and IoT. Consequently, it is illustrated that the duty of CC in IoT functions is the enhancement of applied features. Tao et al. [5] developed a novel multilayer cloud framework to enable efficiency across heterogeneous services that are offered by diverse vendors in the modern home. Also, ontology is included in solving heterogeneity problems that are involved in a layered CC environment. The main aim of ontology is to report the data presentation, knowledge, as well as heterogeneity application that is also used in the security approach to support the security and privacy conservation in interoperations.

Kumar and Gandhi [6] implied a new and reliable three-tier structure to save massive amounts of sensor data. Initially, Tier-1 performs data collection. Secondly, Tier-2 process the large-scale sensor data storage in CC. Finally, a novel detecting technique for Heart Diseases (HD) is developed. As a result, it is carried out with ROC analysis to find signs of HD. Chen et al. [7] applied a new smart in-car camera system that applies a mobile CC method for deep learning (DL). It forecasts the objects from saved videos at the time of driving and selects the specific portions of videos that have to be saved in the cloud for storing local storage space. These models are applicable in attaining optimal prediction value.

Wu et al. [8] focused on developing a novel cloud-centric parallel ML technique for machinery prognostics. It is also employed with a random forest (RF) classifier to detect tool wear in dry milling tasks. Furthermore, a parallel RF method is created under the employment of MapReduce and executed on Amazon Cloud. It is evident that the RF classification model is capable of detecting the exact value. Muhammad et al. [9] performed the monitoring voice pathology of people with the help of CC and IoT. It discusses the possible study of presented voice pathology. Therefore, it is projected with a novel local binary pattern (LBP)–relied detecting system to examine voice pathology inside a monitoring approach. This prediction model attains maximum classification accuracy when compared with alternate traditional methods.

Gelogo et al. [10] defined the fundamentals of IoT with adoptable domains that are accessible in the direction of u-healthcare. This is established with a new technique where it is used in an IoT-centric u-healthcare service. This is helpful in improving the working functions of healthcare care services. Gope and Hwang [11] described a new framework that depends upon IoT medical tools in body area sensors. For instance, a patient could be observed by employing diverse smaller, effective, and lightweight sensors. Furthermore, it is assumed as security requirements for developing the healthcare system. Gubbi et al. [12] explained the vision of structural units as well as upcoming works in IoT technology.

Hossain and Muhammad [13] presented a web observing system named Healthcare Industrial IoT to monitor the patient's health. This is capable of analyzing patients' health data to reduce fatality rate. Therefore, it gathers related patient information that is required to examine the application of sensors and medical tools. But embedded in this model to eliminate clinical errors and diverse risk factors are security modules such as watermarking as well as signal enhancements. Zhang et al. [14] presented different methodologies to develop the applications that are accessible to m-healthcare. These website builders are applied for monitoring the patient's health status under the application of an IoT-centric system. Hence, it has deployed numerous web-relied applications to provide health data of corresponding patients to medical practitioners to provide appropriate treatment. Some other IoT-based healthcare applications are also available in [15–19].

Here, IoT and cloud-based applications are found useful in distinct healthcare applications. To avail prominent e-healthcare services to clients, this chapter presents an IoT and cloud-based disease diagnosis model. A particle swarm optimization (PSO)–based artificial neural network (ANN) called the PSO-ANN model is presented to monitor the diagnosis of the presence of diabetes and its severity level. The application of the PSO algorithm helps to optimize the weights of the ANN model. The data from the benchmark data set and IoT gadgets are used for validation. The validation of the presented PSO-ANN model has been tested using a benchmark diabetes data set. The outcome offered from the experimental analysis clearly pointed out the superior characteristics of the PSO-ANN model over compared methods.

4.2   THE PROPOSED MODEL

The block diagram of the proposed system is depicted in Fig. 4.1. It is comprised of eight major elements:

- Medical IoT Devices
- UCI Repository Data Set
- Medical Records
- Cloud Database
- Data Collection Module

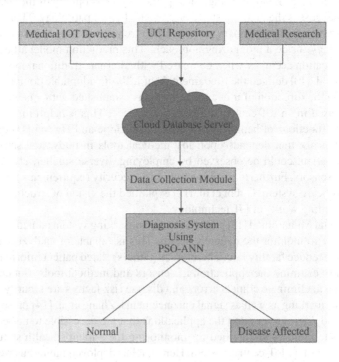

FIGURE 4.1   Block diagram of the proposed model.

- Secured Storage Mechanism
- Health Prediction
- Diagnosing System and Knowledge Base

The wearable as well as the embedded IoT devices are assumed as IoT devices. Such tolls are applied in collecting medical data even at remote sites. The UCI Repository is composed of the diabetes data set. The medical data set contains patient record histories that have been gathered from hospitals. Hence, data sets are saved in the cloud database. The data collection process is suitable for gathering essential data from a cloud database.

The essential data will be saved inside a cloud database for easy access. The health detection as well as the diagnosis is applicable to forecast the disease under the application of the presented classifier method. It is further divided as a subcomponent termed as a severity module that is applied to analyze the disease severity.

4.2.1 DATA COLLECTION

The newly developed CC and IoT-relied on health observing system assumes three kinds of data. It is mainly used in collecting unique patient data that is acquired by applying IoT devices and sensors. Basically, these tools are used for verifying single medical data along with normal data. When an individual medical data exceeds the values of normal data in the case of significant parameters, it forwards an alert message to physicians and to the data collection strategy. Hence, the medical analysis applies 5G mobile networks for sending medical data into a cloud database. In this approach, UCI Repository data set measures can be employed in mapping with original data that is generated by applying IoT devices. Furthermore, clinical medical data can be applied to map with raw data generated with single-patient data.

4.2.2 PSO-ANN MODEL

Here, it is defined as the projected approach for primary prediction and diagnosis of diabetes. In this process, a PSO-optimized NN is employed in the successful prediction of diabetes.

4.2.2.1 ANN Model

Every neuron in the input and hidden layer is linked with one another to the next layer by a few weight rates. The neurons of hidden layers are applicable in computing weighted sums of inputs and include a threshold. The architecture of a multilayer perceptron (MLP) with the help of the input layer, hidden layer, and output layer is applied. Initially, the input layer shows the parameters of data sets. The process of the hidden layer implies the parameters of data sets that cannot be linearly isolated while the output layer gives the required results. Also, a threshold node has been included in the input layer that specifies a weight function. Hence, the simulation outcome is employed in sigmoid activation function. It is represented by Eq. (4.1)

$$p_j = \sum_{i=1}^{n} w_{j,1} x + \Theta_j, m_j = f_j(p_j) \tag{4.1}$$

where p_j shows the linear integration of inputs $X_1, X_2, \ldots, X_n$; threshold Θ_j, w_{ji} implies connection weight among input x_i; neuron j, and f_j signifies activation function; and m_j demonstrates the result. A sigmoid function is a typical choice of activation function and expressed in Eq. (4.2)

$$f(t) = \frac{1}{1+e^{-t}} \qquad (4.2)$$

For training the MLP, the back propagation (BP) learning model is applied, which belongs to gradient descent (GD) model to apply the weights. Each weight vector (w) has been initiated with minimum arbitrary values from a pseudorandom sequence generator, but it is capable of consuming massive steps for training the network, and modified weights are estimated at every iteration. In order to resolve the aforementioned issues, a PSO-centric method has been utilized for evaluating the best value of weight and threshold functions, because PSO is capable of determining optimal solutions.

4.2.2.2   Parameter Optimization of ANN Using PSO

It is pointed out that the weight (w) and bias (b) parameters have a higher influence on ANN function. In this process, the PSO technique is applied for optimizing parameters of ANN. Also, it is one of the populated searching frameworks that is derived from the behavior of bird flocking or fish schooling. It is simple to execute the parameters for modifying. PSO operates a searching function named as a swarm of individuals referred to as particles, which is updated for all iterations. For exploring the optimal solution, every particle migrates toward the direction of the existing best position (pbest) and best global position (gbest). The velocity and position of particles are extended by applying Eqs. (4.3) and (4.4)

$$V_{i,j}(t+1) = W^* V_{i,j}(t) + c_1{}^* r_1{}^* \left(X_{\text{pbest}}(t) - X_{i,j}(t) \right) + c_2{}^* r_2{}^* \left(X_{\text{gbest}}(t) - X_{i,j}(t) \right) \qquad (4.3)$$

$$X_{i,j}(t+1) = X_{i,j}(t) + V_{i,j}(t+1) \qquad (4.4)$$

where t is the iteration value; v_{ij} denotes the velocity of the particle i on jth dimension, where the value is restricted to $[v_{\min}; v_{\max}]$; p_{ij} is a position of the particle i, such that the range $[X_{\min}; X_{\max}]$; X_{pbest} implies a pbest position of a particle i on jth dimension; and X_{gbest} is a gbest position of the swarm on jth dimension.

The inertia weight w is applied for managing global exploration as well as local exploitation; r_1 and r_2 are arbitrary functions from the range $[0,1]$; b represents a constraint factor employed to balance the velocity weight, with the value of 1; positive constants c_1 and c_2 are personal and social learning factors, which have a value of 2; and the particle is comprised of parameters w and b.

Fig. 4.2 implies the task of optimization of ANN parameters using PSO. The major steps of a PSO-relied parameter optimizing task are consolidated as:

Step 1: Initialization

Initially, diverse parameters of PSO are initiated with a population of arbitrary particles as well as velocities.

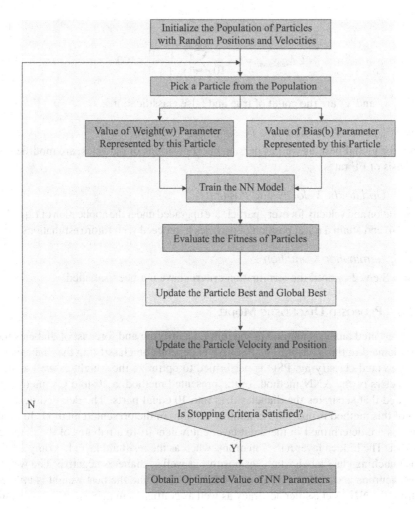

FIGURE 4.2 Flowchart of the PSO-ANN model.

Step 2: Train the ANN Model and Evaluate the Fitness Function

The ANN method undergoes training with parameters c and r from the recent particle. The 10-fold cross-validation (CV) approach is used for evaluating fitness function (FF) values. In 10-fold CV, the training data set has been classified as 10 mutually exclusive subsets with similar size, where 9 subsets can be applied in training the data and the final subset has been utilized for testing 1 data.

The predefined strategy is followed several times such that every subset is applied for testing. The FF is described as $1 - CA_{\text{validation}}$ of the 10-fold CV technique in the training data set, as depicted in Eqs. (4.5) and (4.6). Additionally, a solution that is higher, $A_{\text{validation}}$, would be composed of minimum FF values.

$$Fitness = 1 - CA_{\text{validation}} \tag{4.5}$$

$$CA_{\text{validation}} = 1 - \frac{1}{10} \sum_{i=1}^{10} \left| \frac{y_c}{y_c + y_f} \right| \times 100 \tag{4.6}$$

where, y_c and y_f are the count of true and false classifications.

Step 3: Update the Global and Personal Best Positions

Here, the global best, as well as personal best positions of particles, are modified on the basis of FF rates.

Step 4: Update the Velocity and Position

The position and velocity for every particle are upgraded under the application of Eqs. (4.3) and (4.4) and attain a novel position of particles to proceed with future estimations.

Step 5: Termination Condition

Follow Steps 2–4 until the termination criteria have not been satisfied.

4.2.3 PROPOSED DIAGNOSTIC MODEL

The presented analysis method to the initial identifying and forecast of diabetes has been defined in this section. The PSO-ANN depends on classifying the diabetes. In the presented classifying, PSO is performed to optimize the weight as well as bias parameters of the ANN method. In the presented method, a 10-fold CV method is executed that separates the diabetes data into 10 equal parts. The detailed description of this method is provided in another section. In the presented method, 16 input neurons are determined in the input layer equivalent to 16 attributes of the diabetes data set. The hidden layer has 17 neurons, whereas the resultant layer has only 2 neurons matching class labels: diabetes positive as well as diabetes negative. The weight of all neurons is calculated utilizing the PSO method and the best weight is utilized to train the NN. A classifier accuracy as well as confusion matrix is utilized for estimating the action of the presented diagnostic method.

4.3 PERFORMANCE VALIDATION

Fig. 4.3 investigates the sensitivity analysis of the PSO-ANN with existing models on the applied diabetes data set. The figure ensured that the support vector machine (SVM) model shows its ineffective results with the least sensitivity value of 84.60%. In the same way, it is verified that the naïve bayes (NB) model leads to slightly manageable results with a sensitivity value of 86.40%. Along with that, even better results with the sensitivity value of 91.20% have been offered by the k-nearest neighbor (K-NN) model. Likewise, the decision tree (DT) model has reached a moderate outcome with a high sensitivity value of 93.40%. Simultaneously, the fuzzy neural classifier (FNC) model has obtained near-optimal results with a sensitivity value of 94.50%. At last, the PSO-ANN model has offered supreme results with a sensitivity value of 95.89%.

Fig. 4.4 demonstrates the analysis of the results of the PSO-ANN with existing models on the applied diabetes data set in terms of specificity. The figure ensured

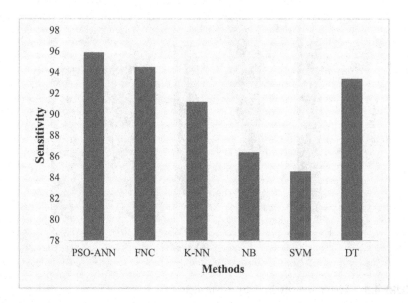

FIGURE 4.3 Sensitivity methods of different techniques.

that the SVM model shows its ineffective results with the least specificity value of 83.40%. In the same way, it is verified that the NB model leads to slightly manageable results with the specificity value of 90%. Along with that, even better results with the specificity value of 93.80% have been offered by the K-NN model. As well, the DT model has reached a moderate outcome with a high specificity value of 96.00%. Concurrently, the FNC model has obtained near-optimal results with a specificity value of 97.30%. At last, the PSO-ANN model has offered supreme results with a specificity value of 98.76%.

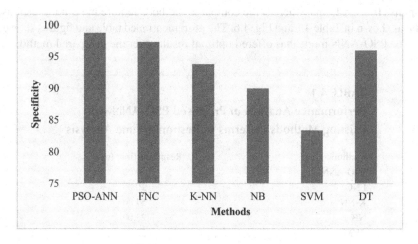

FIGURE 4.4 Specificity analysis of diverse models.

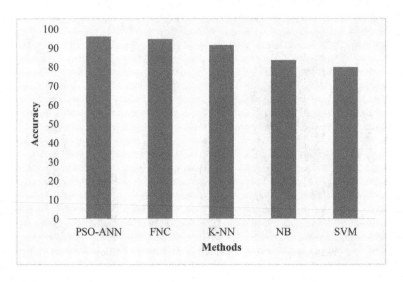

FIGURE 4.5   Accuracy analysis of diverse models.

Fig. 4.5 performs the accuracy analysis of the PSO-ANN with existing models on the applied diabetes data set. The figure ensured that the SVM model shows its ineffective results with the least accuracy value of 80.00%. In the same way, it is verified that the NB model leads to slightly manageable results with an accuracy value of 83.60%. Along with that, even better results with the accuracy value of 91.50% have been offered by the K-NN model. Likewise, the DT model has reached a moderate outcome with a high accuracy value of 93.40%. Simultaneously, the FNC model has obtained near-optimal results with an accuracy value of 94.70%. At last, the PSO-ANN model has offered supreme results with an accuracy value of 96.12%.

Finally, an elaborate response time analysis of diverse models with the PSO-ANN model takes place. It is observed that the PSO-ANN model reaches a minimal response time of 19 ms, whereas the compared methods require maximum response time as shown in Table 4.1 and Fig. 4.6. The aforementioned table and figures showed that the PSO-ANN model has offered optimal results over the compared methods.

TABLE 4.1

Performance Analysis of Proposed PSO-ANN with Existing Methods in Terms of Response Time Analysis

Methods	Response Time (ms)
PSO-ANN	19.00
FNC	20.00
K-NN	57.00
NB	22.00
SVM	32.00
DT	102.00

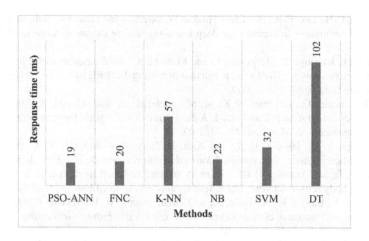

FIGURE 4.6 Response time analysis of diverse models.

4.4 CONCLUSION

This chapter has presented an effective IoT and cloud-based disease diagnosis model. A PSO-based ANN called the PSO-ANN model is presented to monitor the diagnosis of the presence of diabetes and its severity level. The application of the PSO algorithm helps to optimize the weights of the ANN model. The data from the benchmark data set and IoT gadgets are used for validation. The validation of the presented PSO-ANN model has been tested using a benchmark diabetes data set. The outcome offered from the experimental analysis clearly pointed out the superior characteristics of the PSO-ANN model over the compared methods. The proposed model achieves maximum sensitivity of 95.89%, specificity of 98.76%, and accuracy of 96.12%. As a part of future work, the results of the proposed PSO-ANN model can be improved by the use of DL models.

REFERENCES

[1] Emmanouilidou, M. The Internet of Healthcare Things: A European perspective and a review of ethical concerns. *International Journal of Business, Human and Social Sciences*, 13 (5), 675–679, 2019.

[2] Verma, P, and Sood, S. K. Cloud-centric IoT based disease diagnosis healthcare framework. *Journal of Parallel and Distributed Computing*, 116, 27–38, 2018.

[3] Li, Y., Orgerie, A-C., Rodero, I., Amersho, B. L., Parashar, M., and Menaud, J-M. End-to-end energy models for Edge Cloudbased IoT platforms: Application to data stream analysis in IoT, *Future Generation Computer Systems*, 87, 667–678, 2018.

[4] Stergiou, C., Psannis, K. E., Kim, B-G., and Gupta, B. Secure integration of IoT and cloud computing. *Future Generation Computing Systems*, 78, 964–975, 2018.

[5] Tao, M. Zuo, J., Liu, Z., Castiglione, A., and Palmieri, F. Multi-layer cloud architectural model and ontology-based security service framework for IoT-based smart homes. *Future Generation Computing Systems*, 78, 1040–1051, 2018.

[6] Kumar, P. M., and Gandhi, U. D. A novel three-tier Internet of Things architecture with machine learning algorithm for early detection of heart diseases, *Computer Electrical Engineering*, 65, 222–235, 2018.

[7] Chen, C.-H., Lee, C.-R., and Chen-HuaLu, W. Smart in-car camera system using mobile cloud computing framework for deep learning, *Vehicle Communications*, 10, 84–90, 2017.

[8] Wu, D., Jennings, C., Terpenny, J., and Kumara, S. Cloud-based machine learning for predictive analytics: Tool wear prediction in milling. In IEEE International Conference on Big Data, 2016, 2062–2069.

[9] Muhammad, G., Rahman, S. K. M. M., Alelaiwi, A., and Alamri, A. Smart health solution integrating IoT and cloud: A case study of voice pathology monitoring. *IEEE Communications Magazine*, 69–73, 2017.

[10] Gelogo, Y. E., Hwang, H. J., and Kim, H. Internet of things (IoT) framework for uhealthcare system. *International Journal of Smart Home*, 9, 323–330, 2015.

[11] Gope, P., and Hwang, T. BSN-Care: A secure IoT-based modern healthcare system using body sensor network. *IEEE Sensors Journal*, 16 (5), 1368–1376, 2016.

[12] Gubbi, J., Buyya, R., Marusic, S., and Palaniswami, M. Internet of things (IoT): A vision, architectural elements, and future directions. *Future Generation Computer Systems,* 29 (7), 1645–1660, 2015.

[13] Hossain, M. S., and Muhammad, G. Cloud-assisted industrial internet of things (IIoT)–enabled framework for health monitoring. *Computer Networks*, 101, 192–202, 2016.

[14] Zhang, M. W., Tsang, T., Cheow, E., Ho, C. Sh., Yeong, N. B., and Ho, R. C. Enabling psychiatrists to be mobile phone app developers: Insights into app development methodologies, *JMIR Mhealth Uhealth*, 2, 1–8, 2014.

[15] Elhoseny, M., Shankar, K., and Uthayakumar, J. Intelligent Diagnostic Prediction and Classification System for Chronic Kidney Disease. *Scientific Reports*, 9(1), 1–14, 2019.

[16] Lakshmanaprabu, S. K., Mohanty, S. N., Krishnamoorthy, S., Uthayakumar, J., and Shankar, K. Online clinical decision support system using optimal deep neural networks. *Applied Soft Computing*, 81, 105487, 2019.

[17] Elhoseny, M., Bian, G. B., Lakshmanaprabu, S. K., Shankar, K., Singh, A. K., and Wu, W. Effective features to classify ovarian cancer data in internet of medical things. *Computer Networks*, 159, 147–156, 2019.

[18] Kathiresan, S., Sait, A. R. W., Gupta, D., Lakshmanaprabu, S. K., Khanna, A., and Pandey, H. M. Automated detection and classification of fundus diabetic retinopathy images using synergic deep learning model. *Pattern Recognition Letters,* 133, 210–216, 2020.

[19] Raj, R. J. S., Shobana, S. J., Pustokhina, I. V., Pustokhin, D. A., Gupta, D., and Shankar, K. Optimal feature selection-based medical image classification using deep learning model in Internet of Medical Things. *IEEE Access*, 8, 58006–58017, 2020.

5 IoHT-Based Improved Grey Optimization with Support Vector Machine for Gastrointestinal Hemorrhage Detection and Diagnosis Model

5.1 INTRODUCTION

Advanced development of the Internet of Health Things (IoHT) has seen a considerable shift on the way to healthcare technology. IoHT is helpful in the healthcare sector, and is useful for clinics as well as homes. Therefore, there is a requirement for scalable intelligent algorithms, which have resulted in high interoperable solutions and decision-making in IoHT. Wired endoscopy methods are extremely applied for diagnosing and observing the anomalous in the gastrointestinal (GI) tract, such as obscure GI bleeding, Crohn's disease, cancer, and celiac disease. Although it is efficient and stable, conventional endoscopy might cause uneasiness and establish complexities in patients since a longer and flexible tube has to be provided within the GI tract [1]. Additionally, it is tedious to observe the predefined regions of the GI tract, such as larger portions of the small intestine. In addition, the endoscopes require well-trained experts for handling the devices, but also require a longer duration [2]. Finally, technological development as well as effective medical illustrations lead to entirely noninvasive endoscopic systems that do not require sedation, and are available for diagnosing diverse GI malfunctions.

A common Wireless Capsule Endoscopy (WCE) approach is comprised in Fig. 5.1. Alternate capsules apply various sensors, namely, a temperature sensor, pH sensor, and pressure sensor, to evaluate diverse physiological parameters. However, the capsule endoscopy system gains more attention and demonstrates efficiency, but is filled with shortcomings. Some of the constraints are minimized battery-life, poor image quality, absence of localization, and dynamic locomotion controlling.

The task of classifying bleeding and nonbleeding images from WCE images deals with various complications. The battery power of attained final outcome limits the

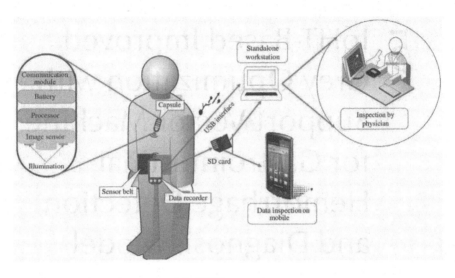

FIGURE 5.1   General structure of the WCE approach.

outcome when it has a minimum resolution of captured frames. Simultaneously, it provides a slower frame value of 2 frames/s. Also, about 6,000 images undergo examination for each iteration. This investigation helps the physician to provide 120 minutes for analyzing an image, which is not applicable to real-time scenarios. Since the validation process consumes a higher duration, the exploring process of bleeding is prone to human fault. Therefore, the automatic prediction method for bleeding frames develops numerous operations for doctors. Suspected Blood Indicator (SBI) [3] is applied to perform the automatic prediction of bleeding frames. However, SBI shows minimum sensitivity and specificity and constantly failed in finding different types of bleeding of the small intestine.

A program deployed with Given Imaging Ltd. allows the physician to look at a couple of successive frames at the same time. Therefore, due to the presence of a minimum rate of the frame, a couple of successive frames do not acquire the concerned area. Consequently, the physician should snap between the images to perform the verification process, which is overburdened and consumes maximum duration. Hence, automatic detecting approaches solve the limitations involved in this model. The primary schemes of GI hemorrhage identification are classified into color as well as texture, and both color through texture-centric methods. The predetermined techniques [4] majorly exploit the ratio of intensity rates in red green blue (RGB) or Hue, Saturation, Index (HSI) domain. The second approach focuses on applying textural data of bleeding as well as nonbleeding images to perform the classification process [5]. It can be clear that a combination of color and texture descriptors provides optimal outcome in terms of accuracy.

The techniques from the initial variety are more rapid, but they do not process the task of finding tiny bleeding portions. The pixel-centric model works on each pixel of an image to produce the feature vectors. Finally, it is comprised of higher processing complexity. The third patch provides maximum sensitivity by giving specificity as well as accuracy. Additionally, the data patch has to be predicted in a manual fashion that conceals the method producing the whole process in an automatic manner. Li and Meng [6] implied a chrominance moment as well as the Uniform Local Binary Pattern (ULBP) approach for detecting the part of bleeding. Hwang et al. [7] signified a super-pixel and red ratio–relied solution that offers good function. Therefore, a high processing cost is observed and it has failed to perform effectively on the images with minimum illumination and better angiodysplasia region.

Few researchers apply MPEG-7 depending on the visual descriptor to find the medical actions [5]. Pan et al. [8] projected a 6-D feature vector used in the probabilistic neural network (PNN) as the classifier. Liu and Yuan [9] presented Raw, Ratio, as well as Histogram feature vectors, which are basically the intensity measures of pixels, and utilized SVM for detecting GI bleeding images. Hegenbart et al. [10] exploited scale-invariant wavelet-based texture features to predict Celiac disease through endoscopic videos. Under the application of MPEG-7 depending on the visual descriptor, a Bayesian and SVM, Cunha et al. [11] segmented the GI tract into four major topographical regions and classified the images. Some other medical diagnosis models were developed in [11–16].

This chapter presents a new Improved Grey Wolf Optimization (IGWO)–based support vector machine (SVM) called the IGWO-SVM model for the detection of bleeding regions from WCE images. The proposed method contains the group of different processes namely data collection, preprocessing, feature extraction, and classification. Once the data is collected and preprocessed, a proficient normalized gray-level co-occurrence matrix (NGLCM) technique is utilized to extract the features from the provided GI images. After that, the classification process is carried out by the use of NGLCM-IGWO-SVM, where the parameters of SVM have been tuned by the IGWO algorithm. The simulation of the NGLCM-IGWO-SVM model takes place using benchmark GI images.

5.2 PROPOSED METHOD

The performance of the proposed method is depicted in Fig. 5.2. The image clearly reveals that the projected approach is composed of a collection of subprocesses. The input GI images are processed for eliminating unknown parts of the image, followed by the computed image applied for feature extracting that extracts only the required features of the image. Finally, a parameter tuning of SVM is carried out under the application of the IGWO model that is applicable for classifying GI images as bleeding as well as nonbleeding areas.

5.2.1 PREPROCESSING

The preprocessing stage is comprised of a group of subprocesses for enhancing the quality of the image and minimizes the speckles without eliminating required features for identifying the task. A median filter has been used to preprocess the GI images. While the preprocessing level is accomplished, the generated image is offered as input for the upcoming level.

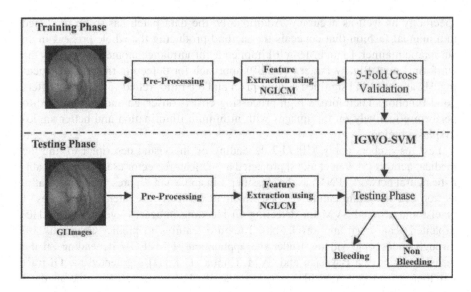

FIGURE 5.2 Block diagram of the NGLCM-IGWO-SVM model.

5.2.2 FEATURE EXTRACTION PROCESS USING NGLCM

To capture the local textural data from image spectra, the collection of different features is carried out from the NGLCM of magnitude spectra of WCE frames. The GLCM is referred as the $L \times L$ matrix of input image, while L is a gray-scale value existing in the images. Fig. 5.3 illustrates the production of GLCM. A couple of successive pixels from an input image is composed with the collection of pixels termed as m and n, which is improved. Under the application of these elements, GLCM has been developed. The location operator P manages the process of interconnecting pixels with one another. In this method, the attained simulation outcome shows that the NGLCM on a frequency spectrum of WCE images are examined.

The creation of the NGLCM performs utilizing Eq. (5.1)

$$N(m,n) = \frac{G(m,n)}{R} \tag{5.1}$$

where R is a pixel pair value in GLCM. NGLCM processes the mapping function for images to a matrix, which refers to the probability of two successive pixel rates. It

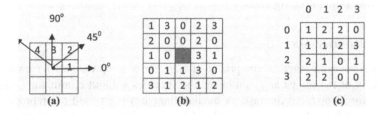

FIGURE 5.3 Generation of GLCM.

shows that NGLCM is composed of local textural data that has to be extracted with the help of images. Additionally, NGLCM -relied texture features are often used in different applications for examining the texture and images. The two features are evolved from the utilization of NGLCM from the projected approach.

There are several types of statistical measures, namely mean, moment, entropy, etc. It is applied to global texture descriptors to validate the complete textual description of an image. After conducting the functions, it can be found that the entropy of frequency spectra provides a productive outcome. The entropy of frequency spectra (E_{fs}) could be written as

$$E_{fs} = -\sum_{m=0}^{L-1} H(z_m)\log_2\left[H(z_m)\right] \tag{5.2}$$

where $H(z_m)$ implies the normalized histogram and L shows a gray level. The randomness of a pixel measure exists in a magnitude spectrum as estimated.

The collection is of 14 features experiments with GLCM-based texture analysis. It cannot be employed with the developed model; it undergoes examination to provide an optimal outcome and is represented as:

1. Contrast (C): It determines the contrast level of grayscale to a closer pixel. The value of C ranges among 0 to $(L-1)^2$.

$$C = \sum_m \sum_n |m-n|^2 N(m,n) \tag{5.3}$$

2. Sum Entropy (S_E):

$$S_E = \sum_{m=2}^{2L} p_{x+y}(m)\log\left[P_{x+y}(m)\right] \tag{5.4}$$

3. Sum Variance (S_V): It estimates the variability of NGLCM dependent on SE.

$$S_V = \sum_{m=2}^{2L} (m - S_V)^2 P_{x+y}(m) \tag{5.5}$$

4. Difference Variance (D_V):
   DV = Variance$[P_{x-y}]$, where P_{x+y} and P_{x-y} is given in Eq. (5.6) and Eq. (5.7)

$$P_{x+y}(k) = \sum_{m=1}^{L}\sum_{n=1}^{L} N(m,n) \quad m+n = k = 2,3,4,\ldots,2L \tag{5.6}$$

$$P_{x-y}(k) = \sum_{m=1}^{L}\sum_{n=1}^{L} N(m,n) \quad |m-n| = k = 1,2,\ldots,L-1 \tag{5.7}$$

Here, an effective local textural feature named Difference Average (DA) can be defined in Eq. (5.8):

$$DA = \sum_{i=0}^{L-1} iP_{x-y}(i) \tag{5.8}$$

Obviously, DA is referred to as $P_{x-y}(i)$. It shows the average pixel values difference in complete NGLCM by considering that the pixel difference is composed of parameters. It will be considered that the feature provides a model about the anticipated pixel difference value of NGLCM. An aspect is vital in texture classification as well as the utilization of automatic detection. The result defines that the presented features exhibit discerning rates from bleeding to nonbleeding frames. The DA is used in classifier textures and other similar applications and residual GLCM-dependent features are carried out.

5.2.3   NGLCM-IGWO-SVM–Based Classification

A GWO technique is inspired by the performance of grey wolves and it depends upon the hunting method of leadership order. A grey wolf is regarded as a top-level hunter and it regularly lives in a group of 5 to 12 wolves. The hunting nature of wolves can be classified into four types: alpha (α), beta (β), delta (δ), and omega (ω). The dominant or leader wolves are known as α wolves that make decisions to choose the place to hunt, sleep, etc. The decisions are made by the α and the other nodes are commanded to follow the orders. The next level of grey wolves is β; they are secondary wolves that use α to generate decisions. The β wolves are considered as α wolves when the α wolves die. The lowest position of grey wolves are ω wolves, which function as scapegoats. When the wolves do not come under α, β, or ω, they are known as subordinate or δ wolves. They are nondominating to α and β wolves, but dominating over ω. The social order is a fascinating nature of grey wolves. The different levels of grey wolf hunting are:

- Approaching victim
- Encircling victim
- Attacking the victim

Here, the hunting process and the social order of grey wolves are defined to design GWO and perform optimization. The GWO algorithm contains exploration as well as the exploitation stage. The former stage searches for optimal solutions in a local explore area. A swarm of grey wolf surrounds and attacks the victim like the process of searching the better results in the local exploration region. The victim is explored in the exploration stage as the victim is explored in the complete explore region. In this procedure of surrounding the victim, the wolf recognizes the place of the victim and surrounds them. Position vectors of the victim are initiate and the explore agents modify the position depending on the achieved optimal result. A surrounded victim is determined as follows

$$\vec{D} = \left| \vec{C}.\vec{U}_p(t) - \vec{U}(t) \right| \tag{5.9}$$

$$\vec{U}(t+1) = \overrightarrow{U_p}(k) - \vec{A}.\vec{D} \tag{5.10}$$

where t indicates the existing round; $\vec{A}$ and $\vec{C}$ are coefficient vectors as well as position vectors of the victim represented as $\overrightarrow{U_p}(k)$; $\vec{U}$ is the position vector; ǁ is the absolute value; and . is element multiplication. Vectors $\vec{A}$ and $\vec{C}$ are defined as

$$\vec{A} = 2\vec{a}.\vec{r} - \vec{a} \tag{5.11}$$

$$\vec{C} = 2.\vec{r} \tag{5.12}$$

where modules of ~a are linearly decreased from 2 to 0 to various rounds and r1, r2 are arbitrary vectors in [0, 1].

A grey wolf has its particular nature of recognizing the locations of the victim and surrounds it. A hunting method is a control with α wolves while the β, as well as δ, can give in any conditions. Additionally, for mathematical reproduction of the pursuing nature of grey wolves, it can be regarded that the α, β, and δ contain more details on the important locations of the victim. Thus, three of the initial results achieved are stored and create another explore agent to inform the position depending on the location of the optimal explore agents that is determined as provided in Eq. (5.13)

$$\vec{D}_\alpha = |\vec{C}_a * \vec{U}_\alpha - \vec{U}|*$$

$$\vec{D}_\beta = |\vec{C}_b * \vec{U}_\beta - \vec{U}| \tag{5.13}$$

$$\vec{D}_\delta = |\vec{C}_c * \vec{U}_\delta - \vec{U}|$$

Where $\vec{D}_\alpha$, $\vec{D}_\beta$, and $\vec{D}_\delta$ are the modified distance vector among the α, β, and γ positions to the other wolves and $\vec{C}_a$, $\vec{C}_b$, and $\vec{C}_c$ are three coefficient vectors utilized in the distance vector.

$$\vec{U}_a = \vec{U}_\alpha - \vec{A}_a * \vec{D}_\alpha$$

$$\vec{U}_b = \vec{U}_\beta - \vec{A}_b * \vec{D}_\beta \tag{5.14}$$

$$\vec{U}_c = \vec{U}_\delta - \vec{A}_c * \vec{D}_\delta$$

where $\vec{U}_a$ is the novel achieved position vectors of α position $\vec{U}_\alpha$ and distance vector $\vec{D}_\alpha$; $\vec{U}_b$ denotes the novel position vector achieved with utilization of β position $\vec{U}_\beta$ and distance vector $\vec{D}_\beta$; $\vec{U}_v$ represents the novel position vector defined with utilization of δ position $\vec{U}_\delta$ and distance vector $\vec{D}_\delta$; and $\vec{A}_a$, $\vec{A}_b$, and $\vec{A}_c$ are three coefficient vectors defined.

$$\vec{U}\,(k+1)=\frac{\sum_{i=1}^{n}\vec{U}_i}{n} \tag{5.15}$$

where $\vec{U}\,(k+1)$ is the novel concluded new position vector, defined with the average total of every position achieved with utilization of α, β, and δ (n = 3). As mentioned, the grey wolves wait to attack the victim until it becomes idle. To model the manner in a mathematical method, the value of ~a is decreased. If the arbitrary values of ~A lie among [−1], the upcoming location of the explore agent is some location separating the current location and the victim's location.

A novel binary GWO (IGWO) is presented to the feature chosen task. Fig. 5.4 shows the flowchart of the presented IGWO. In the IGWO, every grey wolf has the flag vector, whose length is equivalent to the total number of features in the data set.

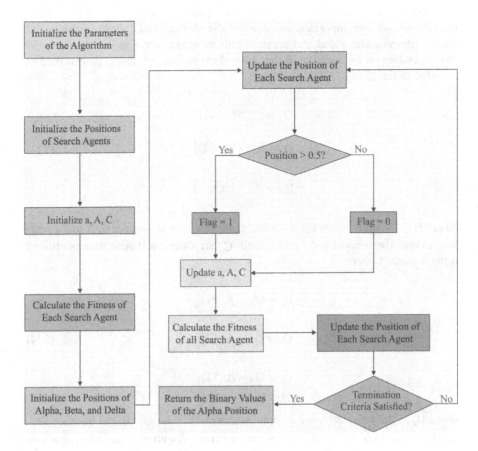

FIGURE 5.4 Flowchart of the IGWO algorithm.

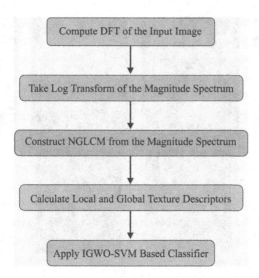

FIGURE 5.5 Flowchart of the proposed NGLCM-IGWO-SVM model.

If the position of a grey wolf were informed with (5.15), the subsequent equation is utilized to separate the position

$$flag_{i,j} = \begin{cases} 1 & U_{i,j} > 0.5 \\ 0 & otherwise, \end{cases} \tag{5.16}$$

where $X_{i,j}$ denotes the jth position of the ith grey wolf.

The proposed NGLCM-IGWO-SVM methodology has two massive stages. Initially, a particle swarm optimization (PSO) is primarily utilized to create the first positions of population, and next IGWO is utilized for choosing the optimal feature group with exploring the feature space adaptively. At the last stage, the SVM classification performed to forecast the classifier accuracy depends on the better feature subset. The flowchart of the presented IGWO-SVM method is represented in Fig. 5.5. An IGWO is mostly utilized to adaptively explore the feature space to the optimal feature group. An optimal feature group is the one with the highest classifier accuracy as well as the lowest number of chosen features. The fitness function utilized in IGWO to estimate the chosen features is the average classifier on the 10-fold cross-validation system.

5.3 EXPERIMENTAL VALIDATION

A collection of simulations is processed to measure the efficiency of the projected method in an empirical fashion. The brief testing diagnosis is carried out in the upcoming sections.

5.3.1 DATA SET USED

A group of around 3,500 WCE images was extracted from a set of 16 bleeding as well as 16 nonbleeding videos taken from 32 patients [17]. These details related to

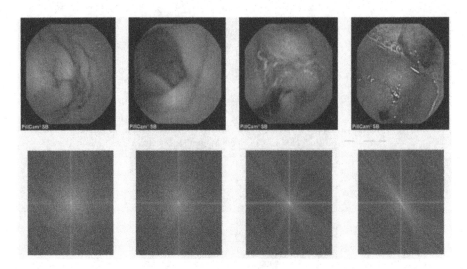

FIGURE 5.6   Sample images with respective magnitude spectrums.

the images are explained here. A similar frame is removed for eliminating the recurrence of images. The noninformative frame is destroyed under the application of remaining food, turbid fluid, bubbles, specular reflection, or fecal content that cannot be removed. By practical applications, it is more significant for classifier bleeding as well as nonbleeding images to the easy access of physicians. Hence, an effective as well as real-time application is capable of resolving the problems involved in frames. All filtered frames from a collection of 32 videos is used to develop a data set. A training data set is comprised with a group of 600 bleeding as well as 600 nonbleeding frames obtained from 12 various people. It can be employed in training the SVM classifier. Simultaneously, the testing data set captured 860 bleeding whereas 860 nonbleeding frames were collected from a residual group of patients. Fig. 5.6 depicts the instance of bleeding and nonbleeding cases. Also, the corresponding magnitude spectrums are obviously depicted.

5.3.2   Results Analysis

Figs. 5.7–5.9 show the results offered by distinct models on the applied WCE images. Fig. 5.7 depicts the comparative study of the applied models in terms of accuracy. It is exhibited that the raw histogram and ratio (RHR) model has resulted in a worse classification of WCE images with a minimal accuracy of 73.72%. In line with, the PNN model has outperformed the earlier model and attained a somewhat maximum accuracy of 74.48%. Along with that, the color moment-local binary patterns (CM-LBP) method has tried to show a manageable WCE image classification outcome and ended up with an accuracy of 77.74%. Concurrently, a competitive classification accuracy of 91.51% has been attained by the super pixel based (SP) model. But, the proposed NGLCM-IGWO-SVM model has resulted to superior classification outcome with the highest accuracy of 92.76%.

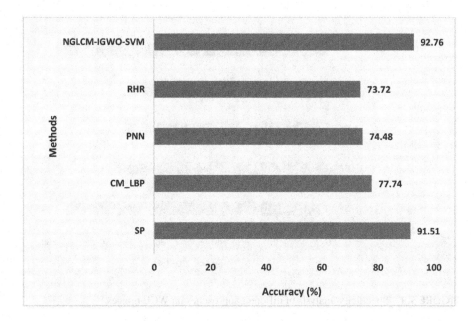

FIGURE 5.7   Accuracy analysis of different approaches on WCE images.

Fig. 5.8 demonstrates the sensitivity analysis of NGLCM-IGWO-SVM model with other models. It is exhibited that the RHR model has resulted to a worse classification of WCE images with a minimal sensitivity of 75.35%. In line with, the PNN

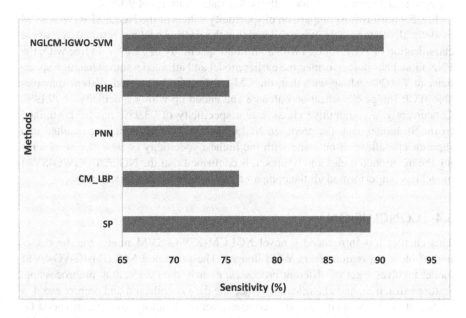

FIGURE 5.8   Sensitivity analysis of different approaches on WCE images.

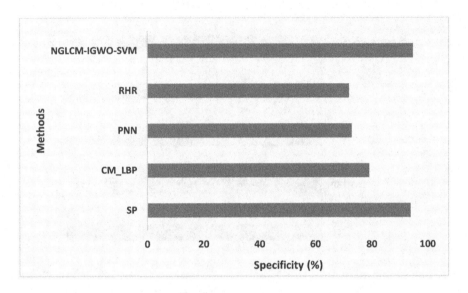

FIGURE 5.9   Specificity analysis of different approaches on WCE images.

model has outperformed the earlier model and attained a somewhat maximum sensitivity of 75.93%. Along with that, the CM-LBP method has tried to show a manageable WCE image classification outcome and ended up with a sensitivity of 76.28%. Concurrently, a competitive classification sensitivity of 89.07% has been attained by the SP model. But, the proposed NGLCM-IGWO-SVM model has resulted in a superior classification outcome with the highest sensitivity of 90.35%.

Fig. 5.9 performs a comparison of specificity values of the NGLCM-IGWO-SVM model with other models. It is exhibited that the RHR model has resulted in a worse classification of WCE images with a minimal specificity of 72.09%. In line with, the PNN model has outperformed the earlier model and attained a somewhat high specificity of 73.02%. Along with that, the CM-LBP method has tried to show manageable WCE image classification outcome and ended up with a specificity of 79.19%. Concurrently, a competitive classification specificity of 93.95% has been attained by the SP model. But, the proposed NGLCM-IGWO-SVM model has resulted in a superior classification outcome with the highest specificity of 94.87%. By observing the mentioned tables and figures, it is confirmed that the NGLCM-IGWO-SVM model has outperformed all the compared methods in a considerable way.

5.4   CONCLUSION

This chapter has introduced a novel NGLCM-IGWO-SVM model for the detection of bleeding regions from WCE images. The presented NGLCM-IGWO-SVM model involves a set of different processes, namely data collection, preprocessing, feature extraction, and classification. Once the data is collected and preprocessed, a proficient NGLCM method is utilized to extract the features from the provided GI images. Then, the classification process is carried out by the use of IGWO-SVM, where the parameters of SVM have been tuned by the IGWO algorithm. The simulation of the NGLCM-IGWO-SVM model takes place using benchmark GI images. The experimental outcome pointed out that the NGLCM-IGWO-SVM model is superior to other models with a maximum accuracy of 92.76%, specificity of 94.87%, and sensitivity of 90.35%. In the future, the NGLCM-IGWO-SVM method could be utilized in real-time applications.

REFERENCES

[1] Emmanouilidou, M., The Internet of Healthcare Things: A European perspective and a review of ethical concerns. *International Journal of Business, Human and Social Sciences*, 13 (5), 675–679, 2019.

[2] Deva, S. V. S. V. P., Akashe, S., and Kim, H. J., Feasible challenges and applications of IoT in healthcare: Essential architecture and challenges in various fields of Internet of Healthcare Things. In *Smart Medical Data Sensing and IoT Systems Design in Healthcare* IGI Global, 2020, 178–200.

[3] Ianculescu, M., and Alexandru, A., Internet of Health Things as a win-win solution for mitigating the paradigm shift inside senior patient-physician shared health management. *International Journal of Computer and Information Engineering*, 13 (10), 573–577, 2019.

[4] Fu, Y., Zhang, W., Mandal, M., and Meng, M.-H. Computer-aided bleeding detection in WCE video, *IEEE Journal of Biomedical and Health Informatics,* 18 (2), 636–642, 2014.

[5] Kumar, R., Zhao, Q., Seshamani, S., Mullin, G., Hager, G., and Dassopoulos, T. Assessment of Crohn's disease lesions in wireless capsule endoscopy images, *IEEE Transactions on Biomedical Engineering,* 59 (2) 355–362, 2012.

[6] Li, B., and Meng, M.-H. Computer-aided detection of bleeding regions for capsule endoscopy images, *IEEE Transactions on Biomedical Engineering*, 56 (4), 1032–1039, 2009.

[7] Hwang, S., Oh, J., Cox, J., Tang, S. J., and Tibbals, H. F. Blood detection in wireless capsule endoscopy using expectation maximization clustering, *Proceedings SPIE*, 6144, 1–11, 2006.

[8] Pan, G., Yan, G., Qiu, X., and Cui, J. Bleeding detection in wireless capsule endoscopy based on probabilistic neural network, *Journal of Medical Systems* 35 (6), 1477–1484, 2011.

[9] Liu, J., and Yuan, X. Obscure bleeding detection in endoscopy images using support vector machines, *Optimization and Engineering* 10 (2), 289–299, 2009.

[10] Hegenbart, S., Uhl, A., Vécsei, A. and Wimmer, G, Scale invariant texture descriptors for classifying celiac disease, *Medical Image Analysis*, 17 (4), 458–474, 2013.

[11] Cunha, J., Coimbra, M., Campos, P., and Soares, J. M. Automated topographic segmentation and transit time estimation in endoscopic capsule exams, *IEEE Transactions on Medical Imaging*, 27 (1), 19–27, 2008.

[12] Lakshmanaprabu, S. K., Mohanty, S. N., Shankar, K., Arunkumar, N., and Ramirez, G. Optimal deep learning model for classification of lung cancer on CT images. *Future Generation Computer Systems*, 92, 374–382, 2019.

[13] Elhoseny, M., and Shankar, K. Optimal bilateral filter and convolutional neural network based denoising method of medical image measurements. *Measurement*, 143, 125–135, 2019.

[14] Shankar, K., Lakshmanaprabu, S. K., Khanna, A., Tanwar, S., Rodrigues, J. J., and Roy, N. R. Alzheimer detection using Group Grey Wolf Optimization based features with convolutional classifier. *Computers & Electrical Engineering*, 77, 230–243, 2019.

[15] Shankar, K., Perumal, E., and Vidhyavathi, R. M. Deep neural network with moth search optimization algorithm based detection and classification of diabetic retinopathy images. *SN Applied Sciences*, 2 (4), 1–10, 2020.

[16] Elhoseny, M., Shankar, K., and Uthayakumar, J. Intelligent diagnostic prediction and classification system for chronic kidney disease. *Scientific Reports*, 9 (1), 1–14, 2019.

[17] Hassan, A.R. and Haque, M.A. Computer-aided gastrointestinal hemorrhage detection in wireless capsule endoscopy videos. *Computer methods and programs in biomedicine,* 122 (3), 341–353, 2015.

6 An Effective-Based Personalized Medicine Recommendation System Using an Ensemble of Extreme Learning Machine Model

6.1 INTRODUCTION

As a new revolution of the Internet, the Internet of Health Things (IoT) is quickly attaining ground as a new research area in different academic and industrial disciplines, particularly in healthcare. Noticeably, because of the advanced propagation of wearable devices and smartphones, the Internet of Things (IoT)–based technologies grow healthcare from a traditional hub-based system to a personalized healthcare system (PHS). A rapid improvement in health data requirements, as well as variations in information, is needed around the world. Based on the study, more U.S. adults make use of the Internet and some users go online to derive health data about diseases, diagnoses, and appropriate remedies [1]. These effects influence the patient–doctor relationship, so that educated patients can easily communicate with doctors [2]. Therefore, patients become more active in making a decision. As a result, the modified way of thinking is named as patient empowerment [3]. However, information overloads, as well as irregular data, are mainly considered to be barriers to attaining results on personal health conditions and necessary actions [4].

In the case of large-scale medical data on diverse channels such as news sites, web forums, and so on, a manifold as well as heterogeneous clinical vocabulary poses an alternate barrier for nonprofessionals [5]. Hence, enhanced delivery of medical context could make users find related data. This medical data is accessible for the patient in making a decision with a dense amount of diverse places [6]. The personal health record system (PHRS) refers to centralizing a patient's health data and enables the owner and authenticated health experts [3]. A recommender system (RS) depends upon the interest of users' details and has evolved in recent decades. A common and familiar one is Amazon's service for products. The main aim of the RS model is to deal with the particular needs of health applications. A health record system (HRS) is an evolution of RS as developed by Kantor et al. [7].

Here, an HRS suggests that the required item is a part of nonconfidential technically approved clinical data that is not connected with personal clinical records. Therefore, an HRS's definitions are derived by individualized health information such as documented personal health records (PHRs). Based on [8], it is a source of data assumed with the user profile of RS. The key objective of an HRS is to provide the user with clinical data that has to be related to the clinical deployment of the patient correlated with the concerned PHR. Relevant medical data might be suggested to health experts with the provided PHR. Also, it is recommended for nonprofessional's inspection of corresponding PHR.

According to the medical expert, HRS must recommend clinical data that becomes more extensive for a patient. The effective combination of a health-based data model is significant for HRSs. As shown in Fig. 6.1, profile-relied HRS units are executed as the expansion of previous PHR technique.

Data entry of a PHR database is comprised of clinical records of PHR authority. The provided medical factor states that an HRS determines a collection of capable items of interest. These items generate from trustworthy health data repositories and might be shown as PHRs online. Hence, it is feasible for computing and offering related data items from secured health-based data repositories. There are two different scenarios as follows.

An RS method is a type of data filtering approach that seeks for predicting fidelity or priority where the user has the desired entity. This is vastly applied in recommending books, videos, and news articles through the Internet. For healthcare application, the RS techniques enclose in making the decision to maintain personal care [9], finding major suggestions between medical experts, exploring preventative healthcare to prepare personalized therapy [10], supplying personalized healthcare assistance, and recommending patients and doctors based on existing consultation records. Widely, it has two types of RS: Collaborative Filtering (CF), which finds the

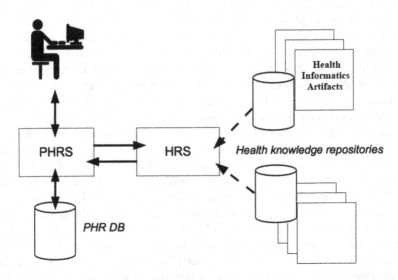

FIGURE 6.1   System context of an HRS-enabled PHR system.

communication among patients and doctors; and Content-Based (CB), which identifies entities for the user as preferred [11].

In particular, CF techniques are employed in analyzing relationships among users and interdependencies items to find priorities affinity over individuals. Matrix Factorization (MF) is applied in familiar realizations of collaborative filtering that tends to scalability as well as domain-free flexibility. MF undergoes characterization in users and items under the application of vectors of secondary features, in which a user's communication with an item is defined by the interior product of latent vectors. Consequently, hybrid methods are integrated with CB and CF models to resolve particular constraints. RS understands regarding user's priorities between items by explicit feedback such as ratings and reviews, while implicit feedback is in the form of presented preferences stated by natural observations. In [12], developers found that problems such as the integration of weak ties and alternate data sources could be applied to uncover identities of peoples from the anonymized data set. Therefore, domains of RSs in health-based medication, remedies, and initial assignment still have ineffective trustworthiness and stability. In point of patients' view, these systems are capable of providing desired suggestions and protect over the worst RS to be more effective. Generally, insurance-based firms as well as healthcare centers focus on enhancing recommendation values by developing capable merit of RS.

This chapter introduces an effective MRS through the use of data mining and deep learning methodologies. The presented MRS involves a set of components, namely database system, data preparation, RS method, model validation, and data visualization. For the RS model, a novel ELM ensemble classifier, namely b-ELM, incorporates the Bag of Little Bootstraps concepts into the ELM.

6.2 THE PROPOSED MEDICAL RECOMMENDER SYSTEM

Here, the RS model has become more valid research in developing artificial intelligence (AI) methods. In contrast, several numbers of RSs aim at e-business, book, and movie recommendation, which offers a virtual experience to apply the proper predictions. As there are higher accuracy and efficiency, it becomes more crucial for online medicine RSs, thus it is estimated with the help of data mining (DM) approaches to attain optimal trade-off from accuracy, efficiency, and reliability. As depicted in Fig. 6.2, the RS framework is comprised of five steps:

1. Database system
2. Data preparation
3. Recommendation system
4. Model evaluation
5. Data visualization

6.2.1 DATABASE SYSTEM MODULE

This module offers data links that are composed with the diagnosis case, drug database, as well as a professional knowledge database. The initial database saves the details of the diagnosis case and gives access to alternate modules. Secondly, the drug database gathers every drug and an index is developed. Finally, experts' knowledge is attained by consolidating professional knowledge.

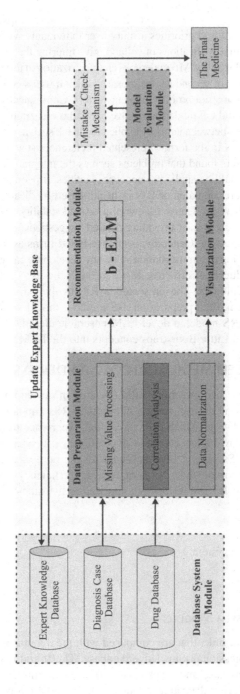

FIGURE 6.2 Overall process of proposed method.

6.2.2 Data Preparation Module

It is treated as a data-cleaner in this approach. A practical data is original, which might be partial and noisy. Thus, data preparation has been created for producing clear information. It is comprised of missing value computation, correlation determining, as well as data optimization.

6.2.3 Recommendation Model Module

This method is deployed under the application of the b-ELM model. Here, it is majorly deployed for building RS on the basis of three techniques. Also, it has been added with novel DM methods to resolve the problems. The visualization module offers visualization methods to project little valid knowledge in diagnosis case data.

6.2.4 Model Evaluation Module

This system estimates diverse RS models in the concrete data set. In the case of a diverse data set, it is required to compute the techniques to attain optimal trade-off between model accuracy, model efficiency, and model scalability. It is assumed to be the overall medicine RS, which uses the DM approaches to medical analysis that complete exploitation of diagnosis case details as well as experts' knowledge. Few RS methods are developed according to diagnosis case data and obtain the drug for an individual integrated with professional knowledge.

6.2.5 Proposed Recommendation Model

6.2.5.1 Extreme Learning Machine (ELM)

ELM is defined as a unique learning model to a single hidden-layer feed-forward neural network (SLFN). The flow diagram, as well as SLFN ELM, is stated in Fig. 6.3 and Fig. 6.4, correspondingly. It is obvious that a diverse gradient-based learning model is applied for normal ANN, the biases and input weights are resolved, and finally, the simulation weights are applied for easy matrix estimations in ELM, and

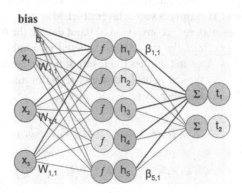

FIGURE 6.3   Single-layer feed forward ELM.

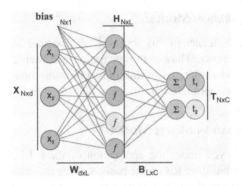

FIGURE 6.4   Structure of ELM.

reducing training duration. Also, ELM is an improvising mechanism from regression applications and massive data set classifying approaches.

Given a collection of N diverse instance $\{(\mathbf{x}\,j, \mathbf{t}\,j)\}\ _j^N = 1$ with inputs $X_j = [X_{j1},$ $X_{j2}, ..., X_{jn}]\,T \in \_\vartheta^n$ and outputs $t_j = [t_{j1}, t_{j2}, ..., t_{jm}]T \in \_\_\vartheta^m$, the ELM with $\tilde{N}$ hidden neurons with activation function $g\,(\cdot)$ is denoted numerically as

$$\sum_{j=1}^{L} \beta_j \phi(W_j X_i + b_j) i\varepsilon[1, N] \tag{6.1}$$

where $W_j = [W_{j1}, [W_{j2}, ..., [W_{jn}]\,T$ is the weight vector that connects the input neurons and jth secret neurons; $\beta j = [\beta j1, \beta j2, ..., \beta jm]\,T$ represents a weight vector from jth secret neurons to resultant neurons; and b_j implies a threshold of jth secret node.

The relation among a target input and output layers of a network is described as

$$Y_i = \sum_{j=1}^{L} \beta_j \phi(W_j X_i + b_j) = t_i \varepsilon i i \varepsilon[1, N] \tag{6.2}$$

The formula can be presented effectively as $\mathbf{H}\,\beta = \mathbf{T}$, where $\beta = [\beta 1, ..., \beta^\sim N]\,T,$ $T = [\mathbf{t}\,1, ..., \mathbf{t}\,N]\,T$ and $\mathbf{H}$ signify a secret layer of ELM.

The hidden neurons undergo a conversion of input data to the diverse presentation as two procedural ways. Initially, the data is detected as a hidden layer by weights with biases of the input layer and implies the result of nonlinear activation functions.

ELMs are resolved as typical neural networks (NN) in matrix form as demonstrated in Fig. 6.4. The matrix form is provided as

$$H = \begin{bmatrix} \varnothing(w_1 x_1 + b_1) & \cdots & \varnothing(w_L x_1 + b_L) \\ \vdots & \ddots & \vdots \\ \varnothing(w_1 x_N + b_1) & \cdots & \varnothing(w_L x_N + b_L) \end{bmatrix}. \tag{6.3}$$

$$\beta = \left(\beta_1^T \cdots \beta_L^T\right)^T, \ \mathbb{T} = \left(y_1^T \cdots y_N^T\right)^T. \tag{6.4}$$

Providing that T shows the target, an exclusive outcome of a system with minimum squared error is identified with the help of the **Moore–Penrose generalized inverse**. Hence, it is computed in an individual process of values in weights of a hidden layer, which tends in a solution with reduced error to predict a destination T

$$H\beta = T \tag{6.5}$$

$$\beta = H^\dagger T$$

6.2.5.2 b-ELM Classifier

Here, it is established with ELM ensemble classification models such as b-ELM. The main aim of using this method is to reach a reliable, effective means of classification in large-scale data. b-ELM applies a Bag of Little Bootstraps (BLB) approach in processing gains as well as productive scalability. BLB is capable of capturing diversities of fundamental classifiers from small subsets. In ELM, training dataset are produced using BLB small subsets for generating the larger original training data set. It makes use of ensemble predictors on training sets, and making decisions and assumed as a detected label. The workflow of b-ELM is provided in Fig. 6.5.

It is composed of two pairs of nested loops in a method: the initial pair of nested loops are employed to find the optimal parameters for base classifiers relied on k-fold cross-validation (CV); the second pair is applied for training base classifiers and obtains predictions for the testing data set. The aggregation stage has a major number of votes to get the final outcome. The parameter $b = n^\gamma$ in technology is a size of subsamples tested with no replacement from the whole actual training data set. Also, $b = n^\gamma$ for $0.5 < \gamma \leq 0.9$. In fact, b-ELM has a maximum favorable space profile when

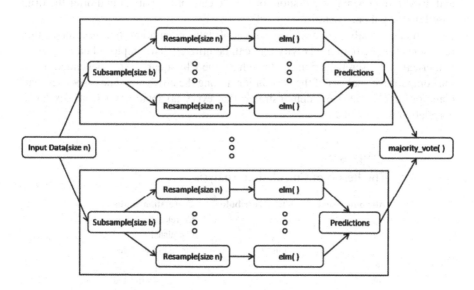

FIGURE 6.5   Workflow of b-ELM.

TABLE 6.1
Attributes of the Diagnosis Case Data

Attribute Name	Attribute Type	Attribute Values
Age	Numeric attribute	15 ~ 74
Sex	Binary attribute	F, M
BP (Blood Pressure)	Discrete attribute	HIGH, NORMAL, LOW
Cholesterol	Discrete attribute	HIGH, NORMAL
Na	Numeric attribute	0.5005 ~ 0.8998
K	Numeric attribute	0.0202 ~ 0.0799
Drug	Discrete attribute	Drug A, B, C, X, Y

compared to Bagging ELM. The parameter s implies a count of subsamples, whereas r signifies re-samples bootstrapped. Therefore, s and r compute the entire number of predictions for the testing data set.

6.3   EXPERIMENTAL RESULTS AND DISCUSSION

Data mining techniques are applied to identify the patterns existing in the data and to get a better understanding of it. The employed data is attained through a technical research website, Data Tang. It holds a total of 1,200 records and the representation of the attributes takes place in Table 6.1. Here, the drug names are denoted by the use of uppercase alphabets, namely A, B, C, X, Y. The numeric attribute represents that attribute values are frequent, whereas the discrete attribute denoting the binary attribute includes a set of two values. The data comprises medical diagnosis data, including age, sex, potassium level, sodium level, blood pressure, cholesterol level, and drug. Fundamentally, a doctor could take care of the patient and offer the drug based on the patient's details.

Correlation analysis is a major process of data preparation, because correlation represents the prediction relativity that can be utilized. The employed data includes numerical and discrete attributes. Therefore, the Chi-square test is dependent upon the comparative analysis of the correlation among the attributes. The associated outcome present in Table 6.2 demonstrated that every attribute apart from sex has a correlation with the drug.

TABLE 6.2
The Result of Correlation Analysis

Attribute Name	Target Attribute	Correlation Status
Age	Drug	Correlated
Na	Drug	Correlated
K	Drug	Strongly Correlated
Sex	Drug	Irrelevant
BP	Drug	Strongly Correlated
Cholesterol	Drug	Correlated

TABLE 6.3

Result Analysis of Proposed b-ELM with Existing Methods

Methods	Accuracy	Running Time
b-ELM	98.54	0.15
SVM	95.00	0.74
BPNN	97.00	1.70
Decision Tree	89.00	0.26

Table 6.3 portrays the results offered by the presented b-ELM-based MRS model in terms of accuracy and running time. Fig. 6.6 shows the accuracy analysis of the presented model over the compared methods. The figure clearly demonstrated that the decision tree (DT) model has offered ineffective recommendations by offering a minimal accuracy of 89%. It is also observed that the SVM model has led to a slightly higher accuracy of 95%. In the same way, it is depicted that the BPNN model has resulted in a manageable outcome with an accuracy of 97% whereas the proposed b-ELM-based MRS leads to a maximal performance with the highest accuracy of 98.54%.

Fig. 6.7 performs a comparison of the response time analysis of the presented model over the compared methods. The figure clearly demonstrated that the BPNN model has offered ineffective recommendation by offering a maximum response time of 1.70 ms. It is also observed that the SVM model has led to a slightly lower response time of 0.74 ms. In the same way, it is depicted that the DT model has resulted in a manageable outcome with the response time of 0.26 ms, whereas

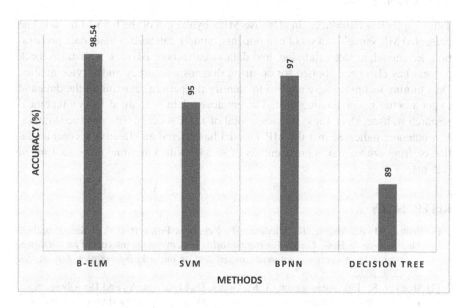

FIGURE 6.6   Comparison of different models in terms of accuracy.

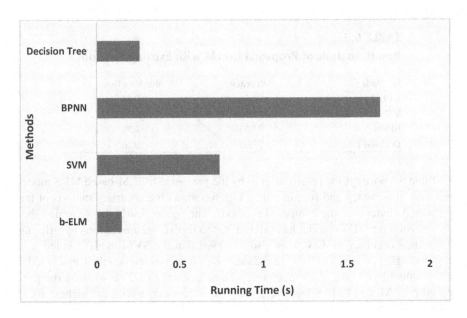

FIGURE 6.7   Comparison of the response time analysis.

the proposed b-ELM-based MRS leads to a maximal performance with the least response time of 0.26 ms.

6.4   CONCLUSION

This chapter has introduced an effective MRS by the use of the b-ELM model. The presented MRS involves a set of components, namely database system, data preparation, RS model, model validation, and data visualization. Besides, a mistake-check process has also been applied for ensuring diagnosis accuracy and service quality. Data mining techniques are applied to identify the patterns existing in the data and to get a better understanding of it. The employed data is attained from a technical research website, Data Tang. It holds a total of 1,200 records. The obtained simulation outcome indicated that the MRS model has offered an effective recommendation of drugs with a maximum accuracy of 98.54% with a minimal response time of 0.15 ms.

REFERENCES

[1] Santos, M. A., Munoz, R., Olivares, R., Rebouças Filho, P. P., Del Ser, J. and de Albuquerque, V. H. C., Online heart monitoring systems on the internet of health things environments: A survey, a reference model and an outlook. *Information Fusion*, 53, 222–239, 2020.
[2] Shankar, K., Lakshmanaprabu, S. K., Gupta, D., Maseleno, A., and De Albuquerque, V. H. C. Optimal feature-based multi-kernel SVM approach for thyroid disease classification. *Journal of Supercomputing*, 1–16, 2018.

[3] Elhoseny, M., Shankar, K., and Uthayakumar, J. Intelligent Diagnostic Prediction and Classification System for chronic kidney disease. *Scientific Reports*, 9 (1), 1–14, 2019.

[4] Raj, R. J. S., Shobana, S. J., Pustokhina, I. V., Pustokhin, D. A., Gupta, D., and Shankar, K. Optimal Feature Selection-Based Medical Image Classification Using Deep Learning Model in Internet of Medical Things, *IEEE Access*, 8, 58006–58017, 2020.

[5] Khamparia, A., Gupta, D., de Albuquerque, V. H. C., Sangaiah, A. K. and Jhaveri, R. H., Internet of health things-driven deep learning system for detection and classification of cervical cells using transfer learning. *Journal of Supercomputing*, 76, 1–19, 2020.

[6] Fernández-Caramés, T. M., Froiz-Míguez, I., Blanco-Novoa, O. and Fraga-Lamas, P., Enabling the internet of mobile crowdsourcing health things: A mobile fog computing, blockchain and IoT based continuous glucose monitoring system for diabetes mellitus research and care, *Sensors*, 19 (15), 3319, 2019.

[7] Kantor, P. B., Ricci, F., Rokach, L., and Shapira, B. *Recommender Systems Handbook*, Springer: Heidelberg, Germany, 2011.

[8] Adomavicius, G., and Tuzhilin, A. Toward the next generation of recommender systems: A survey of the state-of-the-art and possible extensions. *IEEE Transactions of Knowledge and Data Engineering*, 17, 734–749, 2005.

[9] Sezgin, E., and Ozkan, S. A systematic literature review on health recommender systems, in E-Health and Bioengineering Conference (EHB), IEEE, 2013, 1–4.

[10] Graber, F., Beckert, S., Kuster, D., Schmitt, J., Abraham, S., Malberg, H., and Zaunseder, S. Neighborhood-based collaborative filtering for therapy decision support, *Journal of Healthcare Engineering*, 8, 2017.

[11] Adomavicius, G., and Tuzhilin, A. Toward the next generation of recommender systems: A survey of the state-of-the-art and possible extensions, *IEEE Transactions of Knowledge and Data Engineering*, 17, 734–749, 2005.

[12] Ramakrishnan, N., Keller, B. J., Mirza, B. J., Grama, A. Y., and Karypis, G. When being weak is brave: Privacy in recommender systems, *arXiv preprint* cs/0105028, 2001.

7 A Novel MapReduce-Based Hybrid Decision Tree with TFIDF Algorithm for Public Sentiment Mining of Diabetes Mellitus

7.1 INTRODUCTION

In the recent information era, Internet of Health Things (IoHT) objects are embedded in sensors for observing the environment and use an Internet connection for data transmission. It offers the capability of collecting data and examining it in real time. At the same time, due to the development of information technologies, the generation of data becomes higher regularly, which results in establishing a model named "big data." It could be constrained as volume, velocity, variety, validity, and value (5V) [1]. Hence, big data is defined as data that becomes heterogeneous basically and the maximum amount of data has been upgraded with limited duration. It is evaluated that the data produced might be improved to 35 trillion gigabytes (GB) [2]. Big data is massive and robust, and hard to determine when compared with the traditional model [3]. As a result, resolving big data needs diverse methodologies, models, devices, and structures while expanding data at analytical values [4]. In order to deal with developing big data models to produce applicable insight into the latest processing, an analytical approach is essential. Hence, big data analytics is said to be tedious and easy to predict large-scale data that ranges from terabytes (TB) to yottabytes (YB).

Opinion mining or sentiment analysis (SA) through the Internet is assumed to be a novel research field that inspires and produces vital interest between developers. SA is defined as the analysis of emotion toward a product or action [5]. It applied in businesses to point and examine the digital information to enhance the standard of products and provide an optimal service for users [6]. The research on the previous work states the way of developing an opinion and emotions from the attained data by social media. At the initial stage, SA has been employed in classifying movie reviews or product reviews that may be either positive or negative [7]. There are massive techniques in finding sentiment of syntactic, semantic, and feature (machine learning [ML]). The former method applies n-gram [8] and resulted in higher accuracy. The second technique is widely applied by several authors to find the opinion of texts. Most of the research focused on extracting public sentiment under the application of diverse natural language programming (NLP) schemes. Saggion and Funk [9] employed a model to process classification tasks [10]. ML used in identifying sentiment is performed by Zhang et al. [11]; a new ML technique is presented, and feature-based learning is enhanced. Current research aims to know the opinions on social as well as geopolitical content.

The Hadoop Echo system and its elements are typically applied to manage big data [12]. Hadoop is said to be a freely accessible model that enables consumers to save and compute big data in a shared platform over a collection of the system with the application of easy programming modules. It is developed to hold maximum fault-tolerant nature as well as reliability from an individual server to a million nodes [13]. There are three major units of a Hadoop such as Hadoop Distributed File System (HDFS), MapReduce, and Hadoop YARN. HDFS has been created on the basis of the Google File System (GFS). Hadoop MapReduce is said to be a conceptual method at the core of Apache Hadoop to provide numerous scalability in Hadoop clusters. MapReduce can be used in processing more amounts of data. The performance of MapReduce encloses two vital phases such as the Map phase and the Reduce phase. Every phase is comprised of input and output; where input and output job are saved in the file system. This approach follows scheduling operations, tracking, and reimplementing the ineffective operations.

YARN is referred to as cluster managing methodology. It is a major characteristic in second generation of Hadoop, established from knowledge attained from first generation Hadoop. YARN offers resource handling as well as a centralized environment to supply reliable task, secure, and data provisioning devices over Hadoop clusters. Fig. 7.1 depicts the Hadoop platform applied in managing big data effectively.

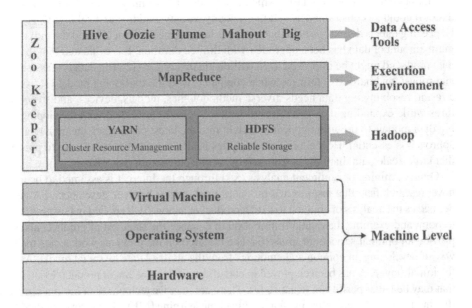

FIGURE 7.1 Hadoop ecosystem.

7.2   THE PROPOSED MODEL

This section defines the proposed system that gathers and examines people's emotions in food, lifestyle, and physical activity with the application of the big data method. It is comprised of three stages: Data Collection, Data Integration, and Analysis.

7.2.1   DATA COLLECTION

The combined, as well as automatic, data models were presented to eliminate large-scale data from different sources. Social network data such as Twitter, Facebook, Blogs, and WhatsApp can be removed on a massive scale by applying an application programming interface (API) provided with diverse social websites as well as Flume, a benchmark big data device employed to eliminate the data. API has the limitation on data controlling value that depends on the time and volume of data eliminated. A modified linear recursive method has been utilized to reject data from large-scale sources. After developing the query, the relevant data is removed and saved in a central memory called the HDFS. Hence, data attained from diverse social websites provide a larger number of parameters as a distinct group. As there is a restriction in India for geographical research, data were avoided to apply the Geo Location accessing data set.

7.2.2   DATA PREPROCESSING AND INTEGRATION

Data that has been eliminated from social media would be a large amount and in an unstructured JavaScript Object Notation (JSON) form, which has noisy and irregular information. Data mining modules such as stop word extraction, stemming, tokenization, and normalization are applied in preprocessing and reject the significant text. Also, MapReduce methods are used for data preprocessing. The data modification is shown in Fig. 7.2.

7.2.2.1   Data Tokenization

Data tokenization is a way of classifying whole information into a set of words with accurate blanks, commas, and spaces. The input data is segmented as words, phrases, useful components, as well as symbols. It is provided as an input for additional tasks. Data tokenization can be operated in two stages: Mode and Characters. Mode tokenizes data on the basis of selected points while Characters segments the data as a specified character.

7.2.2.2   Generating and Removing Stop Words

The stop word creation is deployed under the application of a contextual semantics approach. It is applicable in removing relevant semantics from co-occurrences of tokenized data. Here, the circle is developed with the help of a corresponding task and simple trigonometry is used in determining contextual emotion.

7.2.2.3   Detecting Stop Words with SentiCircles

Stop words in SA are defined as the weak sentiment and the semantics process is carried out. It is comprised of SentiMedian, which is placed in a smaller region

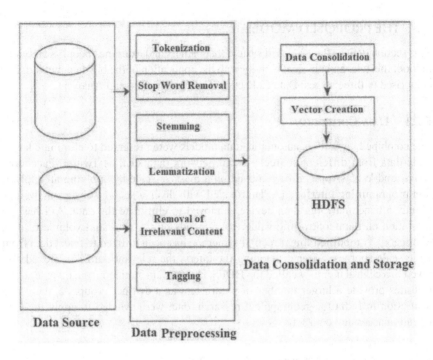

FIGURE 7.2   Data integration model.

closer to the generation of SentiCircle. The points from a site have weak sentiment $d |h| = 0$ and the low correlation is 0. It is useful in finding SentiCircle and computes the whole contextual semantics. The sentiment of SentiMedian guarantees the stop word area. The SentiCircle is used in estimating whole semantics and sentiment with SentiMedian. An edge is applied to terminate stop words regions by the combination of SentiCircle, which has been isolated in the future.

7.2.2.4   Stemming and Lemmatization

These modules are normalized ones that are applied in NLP regions for processing the normalized form. The stemming process is a fundamental estimation; however, it does not give the substitution of the word. The rules generated from the stemming process are utilized for determining stem candidates.

7.2.2.5   Corpus Generation

Corpus is a massive and structured group of text utilized for implementing statistical analysis as well as theory testing. A corpus is utilized for training the classification for identifying positive as well as negative sentiments. The two types of corpus, emoticons as well as user defined corpus, are utilized for classification and identifying emotions of common people. Initially, emotion corpus is applied in classifying data on the basis of sentiment word and icons are used in sentences. The emoticon corpus is composed of linguistical scores to happy emoticons. The next corpus is the semi-automated corpora which is generated by the experts. In addition, the uncommon words are removed and Term Frequency Inverse Document Frequency (TFIDF) technique is used.

7.2.2.6 Tagging

While applying the tag model, the tokenized data will tag under the application of Part-of-speech (POS), Food tag, and external events to analyze the risk issues of diabetes. In the earlier level, text data undergoes tagging by using a Diabetic corpus-based n-gram that varies from maximum ranges. A POS tagging is defined as allocating part-of-tagging speech into words from an input text. Usually, POS implies the tagging of words, enclosed with a slash. Due to the massive data in POS, recent language techniques are applied to the English Penn Treebank tag group problem to tag the social networking data, which performs grouping noise, and unrelated data will be preprocessed.

7.2.3 DATA ANALYSIS STAGE

In this section, the different processes involved in the data analysis stage have been discussed in brief.

7.2.3.1 MPHDT-T-Based Opinion Mining

SA is used for predicting people's attitudes, emotions, opinions, and polarities of a text; which is classified into three stages: Document, Sentence, Aspect level classifiers. For computing the user's opinion from the social network, it is processed by applying MPHDT-T. It is utilized to calculate the polarity of a statement as well as the TFIDF being applied in analyzing the occurrence of words with respect to polarity.

7.2.3.2 Decision Tree (DT)

In this section, the operation of a DT-based classification process along with its sub-processes have been discussed in detail.

7.2.3.2.1 Single Decision Tree (SDT)

The DT classification model employs a tree-like graph structure. Feature vectors are segmented as a single area, equivalent to classes, in sequential techniques. Providing a feature vector, this allocates features for every classifier, in order to make optimal decisions together with nodes that are produced from a DT classifier. By providing a feature vector X, $X \in R^n$, the DT is developed by consecutive phases.

A group of binary questions has emerged, in the form of: $X \subset A$, A subset X for categorical queries, or $X > C_j$ where C_j is the applicable threshold value. For every feature, each feasible value of the threshold C_j determines the particular division of the subset X.

7.2.3.2.2 Splitting Criterion

All binary division of a node creates two descendant nodes if the condition for tree dividing t is dependent on the node impurity function $I(t)$. The different node impurity measures are determined, as represented in Eq. (7.1)

$$I(t) = \phi\big(P(\omega_1 \mid t), P(\omega_2 \mid t), \dots, P(\omega_M \mid t)\big) \qquad (7.1)$$

where ϕ is a random function and $P(\omega_i|t)$ indicates the possibility that vector X_t goes to the class $\omega_i : i = 1, 2, \cdots, M$. The common option to ϕ is the entropy function from Shannon's Information Theory, as represented in Eq. (7.2)

$$I(t) = -\sum_{i=1}^{M} P(\omega_i \mid t) log_2 P(\omega_i \mid t) \qquad (7.2)$$

where log_2 is the logarithm by base 2 and M is the entire number of classes. A reduce in node impurity is determined as represented in Eq. (7.3)

$$\Delta I(t) = I(t) - a_R I(t) - a_L I(t) \qquad (7.3)$$

with a_R, a_L the proportions of the instances in node t, allocated to the right node t_R and the left node t_L, correspondingly. A deduction in node impurity process is defined in Eq. (7.3).

7.2.3.2.3   Stop-Splitting Rule

The easy stop-splitting principle has been adopted if the highest value of $\Delta I(t)$, entirely all feasible divisions, is lesser than a threshold T; after that, dividing is stopped. Another alternative is to stop dividing either if the cardinality of the subset X_t is little sufficient or if X_t is pure, in the sense that each point goes to a single class. The essential factor in planning the DT is its size: it can be large and sufficient; however not too large or else it inclines to learn the specified details of the training set and shows worst generalization action. Studies defined that the threshold value can be used to reduce impurity node by the use of stop-splitting principle, and it does not result in optimal tree size. Several times, it stops the tree developing either too early or too late. The most generally utilized manner is to develop the tree up to a large size initially; after that, prune its nodes based on the pruning condition. Tree sizes are highly essential to the current study as it can be performing a two-class problem. A tree too large or too tiny is inaccurately signifying the feature vectors.

7.2.3.2.4   Class Assignment Rule

After terminating a node, it is assumed to be a leaf and the class label ω_j is provided utilizing the important principle

$$j = argmax P(\omega_i \mid t) \qquad (7.4)$$

Besides, a leaf t is declared to a class where a larger number of vectors X_t go to.

7.2.3.3   Term Frequency-Inverse Document Frequency (TFIDF)

TFIDF is a popular statistical method utilized for classifying text data and indexing the required document. TFIDF is based on frequency and employing a word in a sentence. It is classified under the application of TFIDF to analyze the linked terms for specific diseases from a corpus produced. The TFIDF is determined with the help of Eq. (7.5)

$$td - idf = tf(f_i, d).idf(t_i) \qquad (7.5)$$

where, t_i denotes the ith word, TFIDF of word t_i is sentenced; $rf(r_i, d)$ = TF of word r_i in the sentence; and $idf(r_i)$ is named as IDF. A norm Frequency $rf(r_i, d)$ of word r in the sentence is calculated with word r in sentence d, the Frequency is estimated by Eq. (7.6)

$$tf(t_i, d) = log\left(f(t_i, d)\right) \tag{7.6}$$

IDF is utilized to compute the infrequency of a word in the entire sentence collection. (When the word take paces in every the sentence of the collection, its IDF is 0.)

$$idf(f, D) = log\left(N / Nf \in d\right) \tag{7.7}$$

where N is the whole number of sentences in the corpus; and D and $\cdot Nt \in d$ is the number of terms in that term t is present. The TFIDF is performed utilizing Python in Hadoop Streaming utility as a MapReduce task.

7.3 PERFORMANCE VALIDATION

For validating the effective results of the presented DT-TFIDF model, a data set with varying sizes from 0.28 GB to 1.86 GB on the Hadoop cluster ranging from individual to multiple nodes have been used. The results are examined under varying nodes and data sizes.

Table 7.1 and Fig. 7.3 show the execution time analysis of the proposed model under varying node count and data size. Under the data size of 0.28 GB, the proposed model requires a minimum execution time of 48 s, 50 s, 56 s, and 71 s on 4, 3, 2, and 1 nodes, respectively. Similarly, under the data size of 0.40 GB, the proposed model requires a minimum execution time of 65 s, 79 s, 82 s, and 102 s on 4, 3, 2, and 1 nodes, respectively. Along with that, under the data size of 0.52 GB, the proposed model requires a minimum execution time of 74 s, 83 s, 90 s, and 114 s on 4, 3, 2, and 1 nodes, respectively. Likewise, under the data size of 0.70 GB, the proposed model requires a minimum execution time of 87 s, 100 s, 116 s, and 146 s on 4, 3, 2, and 1 nodes, respectively. In the same way, under the data size of 1.34 GB, the

TABLE 7.1
Execution Time Analysis

Input Data Size(GB)	Exe. Time (s)			
	4 Nodes	3 Nodes	2 Nodes	1 Node
0.28	48	50	56	71
0.40	65	79	82	102
0.52	74	83	90	114
0.70	87	100	116	146
1.34	133	154	176	198
1.86	165	195	213	245

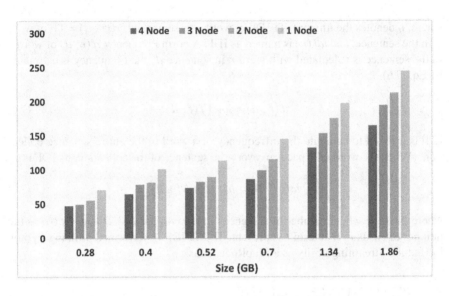

FIGURE 7.3   Execution time analysis.

proposed model requires a minimum execution time of 133 s, 154 s, 176 s, and 198 s on 4, 3, 2, and 1 nodes, respectively. Finally, under the data size of 1.86 GB, the proposed model requires a minimum execution time of 165 s, 195 s, 213 s, and 245 s on 4, 3, 2, and 1 nodes, respectively.

Table 7.2 provides a detailed classifier results analysis of the proposed model under varying n-grams. Fig. 7.4 shows the analysis of the results of the proposed model under unigram. Under unigram, the proposed model classifies positive instances with the precision of 0.76, recall of 0.79, and an F-score of 0.77, whereas the negative instances are properly classified with the precision of 0.72, recall of 0.65, and an F-score of 0.67, respectively.

Similarly, Fig. 7.5 shows the analysis of the results of the proposed model under bigram. With respect to bigram, the proposed model classifies positive instances with the precision of 0.88, recall of 0.81, and an F-score of 0.88, whereas the negative instances are properly classified with the precision of 0.83, recall of 0.89, and

TABLE 7.2

Classification Performance of Proposed Method Using N-Grams

Measures	1-gram		2-gram		3-gram	
	P	N	P	N	P	N
Prec.	0.76	0.72	0.88	0.83	0.55	0.63
Rec.	0.79	0.65	0.81	0.89	0.69	0.56
F-score	0.77	0.67	0.88	0.75	0.72	0.64

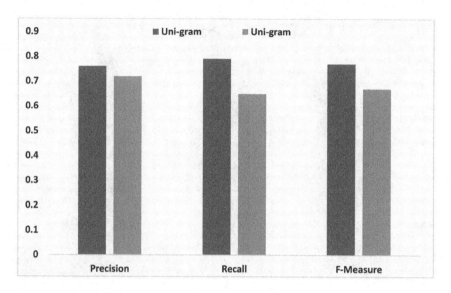

FIGURE 7.4   Results analysis under unigram.

an F-score of 0.75, respectively. In the same way, Fig. 7.6 shows the analysis of the results of the proposed model under trigram. With respect to trigram, the proposed model classifies positive instances with the precision of 0.55, recall of 0.69, and an F-score of 0.72, whereas the negative instances are properly classified with the precision of 0.63, recall of 0.56, and an F-score of 0.64, respectively.

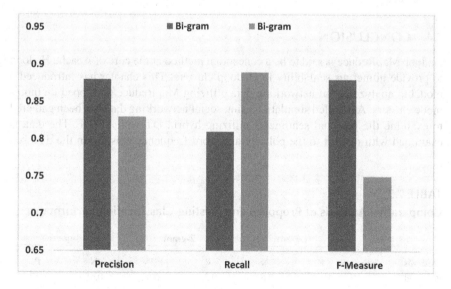

FIGURE 7.5   Results analysis under bigram.

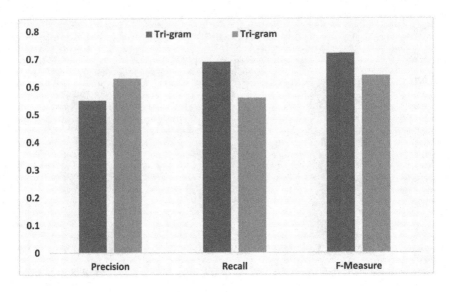

FIGURE 7.6   Results analysis under trigram.

Table 7.3 and Fig. 7.7 depicts a comparative study of the classifier results offered by the proposed model with the Naive Bayes classifiers (NBC)-TFIDF model using n-grams. The comparative study also clearly stated that the proposed model performs well over the compared method in a considerable way.

Although the existing NBC-TFIDF reaches to near optimal values under diverse n-grams, it is exhibited that the proposed model offers superior performance under all aspects.

7.4 CONCLUSION

Hadoop MapReduce is said to be a conceptual method at the core of Apache Hadoop to provide numerous scalability in Hadoop clusters. This chapter has introduced a model to analyze social networking data utilizing MapReduce developed on multi-mode clusters. A detailed simulation using social networking data has been gathered to examine the personal sentiments utilizing hybrid DT with TFIDF. The data is examined with respect to the polarity and word frequency existing in the data set.

TABLE 7.3

Comparative Analysis of Proposed and Existing Classification Performance

Methods	1-gram		2-gram		3-gram	
	P	N	P	P	N	P
Proposed	0.77	0.68	0.86	0.82	0.65	0.61
NBC-TFIDF	0.73	0.64	0.80	0.79	0.61	0.57

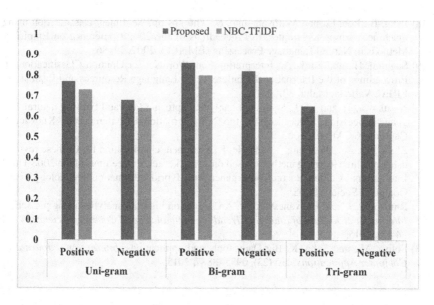

FIGURE 7.7   Comparison of classification results.

The data polarity is determined by the use of DT in terms of 1 to 3 frames. A detailed simulation analysis clearly ensured the effective results of the proposed model over the compared models in a significant way.

REFERENCES

[1] Kang, J. J., Systematic analysis of security implementation for Internet of Health Things in mobile health networks, in *Data science in cybersecurity and cyberthreat intelligence*, Springer, Cham, 2020, 87–113.

[2] Raj, R. J. S., Shobana, S. J., Pustokhina, I. V., Pustokhin, D. A., Gupta, D., and Shankar, K. Optimal feature selection-based medical image classification using deep learning model in Internet of Medical Things, *IEEE Access*, 8, 58006–58017, 2020.

[3] Usak, M., Kubiatko, M., Shabbir, M. S., Viktorovna Dudnik, O., Jermsittiparsert, K. and Rajabion, L., Health care service delivery based on the Internet of things: A systematic and comprehensive study, *International Journal of Communication Systems*, 33(2), e4179, 2020.

[4] Elhoseny, M., Bian, G. B., Lakshmanaprabu, S. K., Shankar, K., Singh, A. K., and Wu, W. Effective features to classify ovarian cancer data in internet of medical things, *Computer Networks*, 159, 147–156, 2019.

[5] Marlen, K., Tien, D. H., and Nikos, D., Twitter data analysis for studying communities of practice in the media industry, *Telematics Information*, 35 (1), 195–212, 2018.

[6] Lakshmanaprabu, S. K., Mohanty, S. N., Krishnamoorthy, S., Uthayakumar, J., and Shankar, K. Online clinical decision support system using optimal deep neural networks, *Applied Soft Computing*, 81, 105487, 2019.

[7] Elhoseny, M., and Shankar, K. Optimal bilateral filter and convolutional neural network based denoising method of medical image measurements, *Measurement*, 143, 125–135, 2019.

[8] Pang, B., Lee, L., and Vaithyanathan, S., Thumbs up? Sentiment classification using machine learning techniques, in Proceedings of the 2002 Conference on Empirical Methods in Natural Language Processing (EMNLP), 2002, 79–86.

[9] Saggion, H., and Funk, A., Interpreting SentiWordNet for Opinion Classification, in Proceedings of the International Conference on Language Resources and Evaluation, LREC, Valletta, Malta, 2010.

[10] Nasukawa, T., and Yi, J., Sentiment analysis: capturing favorability using natural language processing, Proceedings of the 2nd International Conference on Knowledge Capture, K-CAP '03, 2003.

[11] Zhang, C., Zuo, W., Peng, T., and He, F., Sentiment classification for Chinese reviews using machine learning methods based on string kernel, Proceedings of the 2008 Third International Conference on Convergence and Hybrid Information Technology, IEEE Computer Society, 2008.

[12] Ramsingh, J., and Bhuvaneswari, V. An insight on big-data analytics using pig script, *International Journal of Emerging Trends in Technology and Computer Science*, 4 (6), 84–90, 2015.

[13] Sofiya, M., and Soha, K. Big Data: tools and applications, *International Journal of Computer Applications*, 115 (23), 0975–8887, 2015.

8 IoHT with Artificial Intelligence–Based Breast Cancer Diagnosis Model

8.1 INTRODUCTION

The Internet of Health Things (IoT) is defined as the collection of intelligent healthcare devices that are associated with one another and interchange patient data using the Internet. Such models are applied for detecting diverse healthcare issues, to execute the approach that has been used for predicting several diseases. Tumors, a type of malady and strategy of breast cancer disease, are a mild growth of cells in specific regions of the body. Breast malignancy is structured while the disease is developed from tissue [1]. Based on the survey of the World Social Insurance Association, there is a rapid improvement of breast cancer disease globally [2]. The earlier identification of tumor helps to increase the survival rate. A mammography is employed for initial analysis, location, as well as a remedy of breast cancer. Regular mammograms are the better ways to determine the breast cancer in the earlier time. Breast imaging of mammography is carried out using minimum values of Xbeams with higher goals as well as maximum differentiation [3–5].

Here, full field advanced mammography (FFDM) has been used to eliminate superfluous biopsies. Due to the large enquiries regarding particular applications, it is required for developing a processing approach to trigger the radiologist. These models are capable of providing well-equipped data and extending the correct recognition values for diseases such as breast cancer. Hence, the breast cancer diagnosis has the ability to determine the affected regions clearly. A breast malignancy computer-aided diagnosis (CAD) approach results in assisting imperative as well as being vital for breast growth management. A mammography offers the philosophy to assist the radiologist to predict wider mammogram pictures and classify as normal and abnormal [6]. Similarly, it distinguishes cell growth as a minimum and maximum. Recently, multiple classifications of therapeutic results have been carried out. It provides the likelihood of errors and results within a wider time frame. The model's implementation depends upon techniques applied for the classification of mammogram images as well as highlighting the extraction point. Benchmark enhancement models such as histograms are used in an intrigued region of the mammogram image. Complexity extension is performed among the region of intrigue as well as close-by typical tissue.

Breast cancer has been assumed as rapidly extended malignancy in women of Western nations and developed urban communities in India [7]. The American

Cancer Society reports that 1 in 8 women (about 12%) in the United States would be computed to have breast cancer. Mammography, biopsy, and biopsy needle, are three principles for common recognition of a breast tumor. The primary phase is a mammography for analyzing the breast tumor. The mammogram has the ability to determine the tumor region created by malicious cells and disease results in tumor delivered by the carcinogenic cell. The current application of textural methods as well as the machine learning (ML) classification has been developed with alternate analysis, which leads to realizing the breast malignancy. Several experts applied specific region of interest (ROI) for surface analysis. ROI in a mammogram image has been classified as a possible number of nonoverlapping tiny squared shaped regions of permanent size to require a higher data set for future studies. A common mammogram classification is often classified as three sequential phases: (1) extraction of ROI, (2) feature extraction from the desired ROI, and (3) classifying mammogram features.

This chapter defines the principles for classification as well as feature extraction. In this approach, hybrid feature extraction (HFE) is applied for predicting features of mammogram images and undergoes classification of applying genetic algorithm with support vector machine (GA-SVM). The classification accuracy is maximum under the application of the GA-SVM classifier. It is clear that the presented system efficiently categorizes abnormal mammograms.

8.2   RELATED WORKS

Different techniques have been implemented by the developers of breast cancer segmentation as well as classification. Here, an extensive estimation of some required contributions to previous studies is proposed. Abubacker et al. [8] implied a productive classifier under the application of the Genetic Association Rule Miner (GARM) and neural network (NN). A multivariate filter has been applied to eliminate the proper feature values that tend to improve the accuracy of classification. Wider implementations were executed out on the MIAS database to show the robust form of the projected model. Some of the demerits of GARM-NN technology were highly tedious to identify the free space. Free space is capable of providing optimal discriminant features.

Kumar et al. [9] applied a hybrid hierarchical technique to classify the density of breast cancer with the application of electronic mammogram pictures. There are about four categories of breast density, which are implemented by applying hybrid hierarchical methods. Dora et al. [10] proposed novel models, such as the Gauss–Newton presentation with a sparse depiction of breast cancer prediction. The deployed method is comprised of two main benefits: minimum response time as well as lower processing complexity associated with alternate traditional sparse approaches. Zaher and Eldeib [11] implemented a novel unsupervised breast cancer prediction model applying the Deep Belief Network (DBN) with a supervised back propagation (BP) technique. The executed approach has been built using the Liebenberg Marquardt learning function for initializing the weight of DBN.

Cong et al. [12] projected a selective method to diagnose breast cancer from ultrasound as well as mammogram images. A selective methodology has been combined with classifications like *k*-nearest neighbor (K-NN), SVM, and Naive Bayes (NB) to analyze breast cancer. The integrated classifications were effective in breast cancer prediction, which attained higher accuracy as well as sensitivity related to a single classification model. This study shows evidence that classifier-integration is more optimal when compared with the feature-fusion approach in every factor while the deployed classifier-fusion technique fails the development of cancer cell boundaries, which is comprised.

Wang et al. [13] developed a microwave breast cancer analyzing method to detect the numerical breast phantoms that are based on weighted T1 and T2, which undergoes distortion. A similar grid undergoes mapping with sane dielectric features of tissues under the application of the edge detection calibration method as well as tissue deviation masks. The simulation outcome of grids is mapped with dielectric features under the application of piecewise-linear matching. Hence, a deployed model functions more effectively when compared with previous models that predict the portions of mammograms such as realistic skin, chest wall, and so on. It is applicable in 2D mammogram images and not for 3D images. Some other models for disease diagnosis are also found in the literature [14–18].

8.3   THE PROPOSED MODEL

Fig. 8.1 shows the working process of the proposed model. The mammograms are said to be preprocessed images at the primary stage and improve the variations among objects as well as irregular background noise. Intensity is one of the parameters

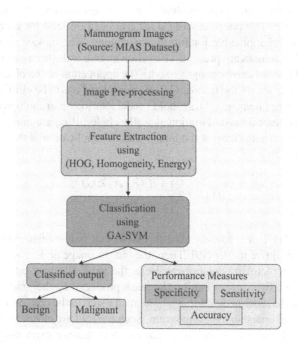

FIGURE 8.1   Overall process of proposed method.

calculated in this approach. Preprocessing is carried out due to the minimum contrast of mammographic pictures, which is very complex to interrupt the masses present in a mammogram image. In general, there is no vast difference in the severity of pectoral muscle than tumor intensity. Thus, it tends to eliminate the pectoral muscle region before processing the feature extraction. The preprocessing phase is more applicable in eliminating labels and background noise present in electronic mammograms. Once the unwanted labels and noise were removed from a mammogram, the feature extraction stage has been used in a computed image that is the same as random transform. Therefore, it is majorly employed in predicting random arbitrary shapes as well as straight lines. These features are extracted efficiently and isolated. Consequently, GA-SVM has been applied for classification operation.

8.3.1 IMAGE ACQUISITION

A mammogram image can be normal, benign, and malignant in the case of fatty-glandular breast types that have been gathered from the MIAS database for predicting the disease. It is comprised of mammogram images at a 50-mm pixel edge. It is applied where images are 1024 × 1024 pixels. Around 300 mammogram images derived from 94 images have been deployed for this task. Cancer detection is complex to identify in the mammogram. Hence, dense images cannot be applied to the analyzing process.

8.3.2 PREPROCESSING

The images gathered from the database are composed of irregular data as well as background noise. The preprocessing stage has been utilized for eliminating such mammograms and applicable for future experiments. The unwanted area of breast cancer as well as tumors are present. The yellow region is the breast region; irregular label and background can be projected with the application of the blue circle as well as a red circle that shows the tumor. The unknown label has to be eliminated initially by applying the gradient relied threshold model. Various morphological tasks were processed to produce a mask. Dilation as well as hole-filling are major tasks applied to produce a binary edge map of the image with the application of the gradient relied threshold approach.

$$f(x,y) = \begin{cases} 1 \ if \ G(x,y) \geq GT \\ 0 \ else \end{cases} \qquad (8.1)$$

In this model, GT is a gradient-based threshold that is identified with the application of Otsu's adaptive model [19]. Then, the binary image undergoes dilations with the help of the structuring component. Here, the mask is improved with the actual image. The given two images exhibit the mask produced by the gradient model and the alternate is the label-avoided image. The major step in the next process is to eliminate the pectoral image in a mammogram. Such muscles are closer to intensity value when compared with tumor intensity. For effective feature extraction process, the unwanted regions are needed to the removed by the use of segmentation techniques.

8.3.3 HFE Model

In the presented approach, hybrid feature extraction has experimented with converted mammogram images. Here, a higher-level feature, termed as the Gray-Level Co-occurrence Matrix (GLCM), is applied to extract the features of mammogram images. There are two productive GLCM texture features that were assumed: homogeneity and power. Additionally, the histogram of oriented gradients (HOG) descriptor has been utilized in medical image processing as well as computer vision to extract optimized feature values. A wider definition of HOG and GLCM texture features are explained in upcoming sections.

8.3.3.1 Homogeneity

Homogeneity computes distribution units in the GLCM. To quantitatively simplify the homogeneous texture for affinity, the local spatial statistics of texture has been determined under the application of scale as well as orientation selection of Gabor filtering. These mammogram images are further divided as a collection of homogeneous texture and texture features are relevant to regions of subjected image data. In GLCM, homogeneity operates on four directions such as $\theta = 0°$, $45°$, $90°$, or $135°$ with a feature vector size of 4. It provides maximum accuracy to detect the infected regions that are defined using the vulnerable difference in gray level. A typical formula to determine the homogeneity is expressed in Eq. (8.2)

$$Homogeneity = \sum_{i=0}^{n-1}\sum_{j=0}^{n-1} \frac{P_{ij}}{1+(i-j)^2} \tag{8.2}$$

8.3.3.2 Energy

Energy is used to measure the uniformity of normalized pixel pair distributions and computes the number of duplicate pairs. Energy is defined as a normalized value with a higher range of 1. The higher energy value exists if the gray level distribution has a regular format. Energy is applicable in reflecting depth as well as the smoothness of mammogram images. The typical expression of computing energy of the mammogram image is provided in Eq. (8.3)

$$Energy = \sum_{i=0}^{n-1}\sum_{j=0}^{n-1} -\ln(P_{ij})P_{ij} \tag{8.3}$$

where n denotes the gray levels, $P(i, j)$ implies the pixel value of position (i, j) of mammogram images, and P_{ij} signifies a normalized co-occurrence matrix.

8.3.3.3 HOG Features

The main feature in the HOG descriptor can hold the local appearance of objects and account the invariance of object conversions, as well as illumination status as the edge and data regarding gradients are estimated by using a multiple coordinate-HOG feature vector. Initially, a gradient operator N has been applied to determine the gradient measure. The gradient point of the mammogram image is presented as

G and image frames are shown as I. A common formula used in computing gradient points is provided in Eq. (8.4)

$$G_x = N * I(x,y) \text{ and } G_x = N^T * I(x,y) \qquad (8.4)$$

The image-detecting window undergoes characterization as diverse spatial regions that are named as cells. Therefore, the magnitude gradients of pixels are implemented with edge orientation. As a result, the magnitude of gradients (x, y) is implied in Eq. (8.5)

$$G_x(x,y) = \sqrt{G_x(x,y)^2} + \sqrt{G_y(x,y)^2} \qquad (8.5)$$

The edge orientation of point (x, y) is provided in Eq. (8.6)

$$\theta(x,y) = \tan^{-1} \frac{G_y(x,y)}{G_x(x,y)} \qquad (8.6)$$

where Gx represents the horizontal direction of gradients and Gy denotes the vertical direction of gradients. The graphical architecture of the HOG descriptor is provided in Fig. 8.2. In case of enhanced illumination as well as noise, a normalization task is processed once completing the histogram measures. The determination of normalization is used in contrast and local histograms can be validated. In multiple coordinate HOG, four diverse approaches of normalization can be applied such as L2-norm, L2-Hys, L1-Sqrt, and L1-norm. When compared to this normalization, L2-norm provides an optimal function in cancer prediction. The segments of normalization in HOG are expressed in Eq. (8.7)

$$L2 - \text{norm} : f = \frac{h}{\sqrt{\| h \|_2^2 + e^2}} \qquad (8.7)$$

where e implies a small positive value used in regularization, f can be a represented feature vector, h shows the nonnormalized vector, and $\| h \|_2^2$ is named as 2-norm of HOG normalization.

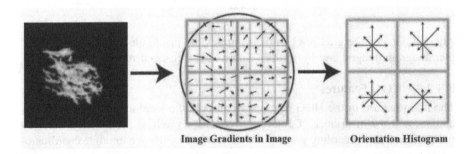

Image Gradients in Image   **Orientation Histogram**

FIGURE 8.2   Representation of the HOG descriptor.

8.3.4 GA-SVM-BASED CLASSIFICATION

A GA can be an effective classification as well as a parameter optimization relevant to the development of chromosomes, estimation of fitness function (FF), and system process and is represented in upcoming sections.

8.3.4.1 Chromosome Design

An SVM classifier with a radial basis function (RBF) kernel is used in classifying land-cover classes; however, the parameters C and γ are estimated. Hence, the chromosome is constrained in three portions: the selected features, C, and γ. A binary coding model has been used to compute the chromosome. The features are deployed as $Fb_1 \sim Fb_{nf}$, which implements input features; $Fb_i = 1$, if a corresponding feature has been selected; and $Fb_i = 0$, if a feature has not been selected. $Cb_{1b} \sim Cb_{nc}$ is a value of C, and $\gamma b_1 \sim \gamma b_{ny}$ is a measure of γ. The norm nf is referred to as a number of bits showing the features, nc denotes the number of bits the parameter C, and $n\gamma$ implies the count of bits showing the parameter γ.

8.3.4.2 Fitness Function

It is one of the major portions of estimating whether an individual can "fit" to live to produce the units. It is applied with two strategies to describe the FF such as the classifying accuracy as well as several features from a selected subset. When an individual is comprised of maximum classification accuracy and minimum features, the function has greater high fitness measure and maximum probability to pass in the upcoming generation, as provided in Eq. (8.8)

$$Fitness = W_{OA} \times OA_{SVM} + \left(W_f . \frac{\sum\nolimits_{nf}^{i=1} f_i}{n_f} \right) \tag{8.8}$$

where W_{OA}, OA_{SVM}, W_f and f_i implies the weight of classification accuracy, overall classifier accuracy, feature weights, as well as mask value. Here, it is computed with FF of classification accuracy weight (W_{OA}) and weight of features (W_f) of 0.2 for every data set.

8.3.4.3 Hybridization of the GA-SVM Algorithm

The major function in GA-based feature selection (FS), as well as parameter optimizing, is consolidated here.

- Chromosomes present from the initial population, such as feature subset as well as SVM kernel parameters (C, γ), are produced. The basic size of the population has to be selected by the customer.
- The FF values of all chromosomes such as C, γ, and the chosen feature subset are computed.
- In the SVM classifier, the training, as well as testing samples of every class retrieved from ROI, are employed according to professional interpretation. In case of the training set, a combined image was used in training the SVM

classification, and testing samples were used in assessing the classification accuracy.

- Fitness values of individuals are calculation with the application FF, and based on classification accuracy as well as selected features.
- Individuals with higher fitness measures would be selected and provisioned for the next generation in genetic operation procedures.
- When a termination condition is met, the process terminates at best individuals. Hence, the normalized outcomes are comprised of C, γ, and selected features. Otherwise, the process would be repeated with the next generation under the application of genetic task, such as selection, crossover, as well as mutation.

8.4 PERFORMANCE VALIDATION

For simulation purposes, the MIAS data set has been validated for assessing the results of the proposed model. Among the total number of images, a set of 80% of images was used for training and 20% of images were used for testing. Fig. 8.3 shows the sample set of benign and malignant images.

Fig. 8.4 shows the visualization outcome of the proposed model. In Fig. 8.4a, the white circle shows the unwanted objects in the mammogram image, the red circle indicates the tumor masses present in the image, and the yellow circle denotes the normal image. Fig. 8.4b indicates the binary form of the applied input image and Fig. 8.4c represents the preprocessed image.

Fig. 8.5 shows the sensitivity analysis of diverse models on the applied MIAS data set. It is shown that the Energy-NB model has provided a minimum sensitivity of 26.40%. Next to that, the hybrid features-NB model has offered a slightly higher sensitivity of 28%. Along with that, the homogeneity-NB model has provided a sensitivity value of 32%. At the same time, the Homogeneity-SVM, HOG-NN, HOG-NB, and HOG-DNN models lead to moderate and near-identical results of 37.60%, 38.40%, 38%, and 38.40%, respectively. In the same way, the Homogeneity-NN and Homogeneity-DNN models reach an acceptable sensitivity of 54.40%. Besides, it is noted that the Energy-NN, Energy-DNN, HOG-SVM, Hybrid Features-NN, and Hybrid Features-SVM models provide manageable results with the sensitivity values of 56.80%, 56.80%, 57.60%, 58.40%, 58%, and 58.40%. Likewise, it is observed that the Energy-SVM model leads to a higher sensitivity value of 69.60%. At last, the proposed Hybrid features-GA-SVM model has resulted in a maximum sensitivity value of 72.56%.

Fig. 8.6 exhibits the specificity analysis of various methods on the used MIAS data set. It is expressed that the HOG-SVM method has given a minimum specificity of 32.80%. Then, the Energy-SVM approach has provided a slightly higher specificity of 38.80%. In line with this, the homogeneity-NN model has offered a specificity of 39.20%. Simultaneously, the HOG-NB and Hybrid Features-SVM models tend to a gradual and near-identical results of 47.20% and 48.40%, correspondingly. Likewise, the Energy-NN, Homogeneity-DNN, HOG-NN, and HOG-DNN models attain to an acceptable specificity of 56.40%, 59.20%, 53.60%, and 55.60%, respectively. On the other hand, the Energy-NN, Energy-DNN, HOG-SVM, Hybrid Features-NN,

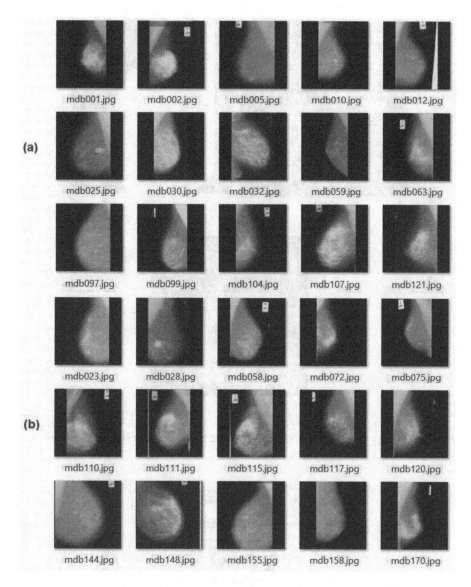

FIGURE 8.3   Sample images: (a) benign, (b) malignant.

and Hybrid Features-SVM models provide acceptable results with the specificity of 56.80%, 56.80%, 57.60%, 58.40%, 58%, and 58.40%, correspondingly. Similarly, it is pointed out that the Energy-NB and Homogeneity models lead to a maximum specificity value of 74% and 72%, respectively. Finally, the proposed Hybrid features-GA-SVM model has concluded to a higher specificity value of 78.34%.

Fig. 8.7 defines the accuracy analysis of various methodologies on the applied MIAS data set. It is provided that the HOG-NB model has given a lower accuracy of

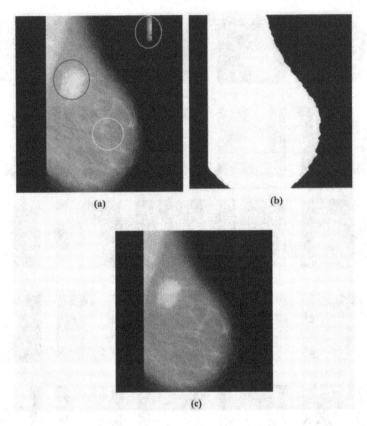

FIGURE 8.4 (a) Original image, (b) label removed binary image, (c) preprocessed image.

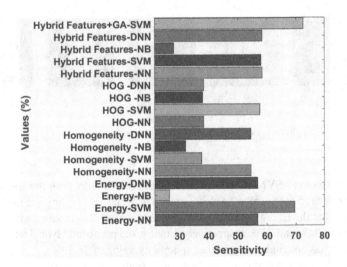

FIGURE 8.5 Sensitivity analysis of diverse models.

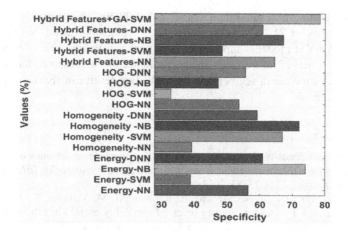

FIGURE 8.6   Specificity analysis of diverse models.

42.60%. In line with this, it is noted that the Hybrid Features-DNN model leads to a maximum accuracy value of 59.60%. Consequently, the proposed Hybrid features-GA-SVM technique has resulted in a higher accuracy value of 74.28%. These values showcased that the Hybrid features-GA-SVM model is qualified to alternate models in a significant way.

8.5   CONCLUSION

This chapter has presented an effective IoT-based Breast Cancer Diagnosis using the Hybrid Features-GA-SVM model. The proposed model involves a set of different stages namely image acquisition, preprocessing, HFE process, and GA-SVM-based classification. The proposed model has been tested using a benchmark MIAS data set. The experimental outcome ensured that the Hybrid Features-GA-SVM

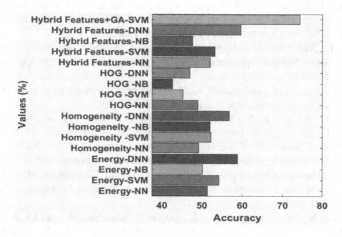

FIGURE 8.7   Accuracy analysis of diverse models.

model has resulted in a maximum sensitivity of 72.56%, a specificity of 78.34%, and an accuracy of 74.28%, respectively. These values portrayed that the Hybrid Features-GA-SVM model is superior in breast cancer classification over compared methods. As a part of future work, the performance of the presented technique can be increased by the use of segmentation models. Besides, it can also be employed in real-time diagnosis.

REFERENCES

[1] He, D., and Zeadally, S. An analysis of RFID authentication schemes for Internet of Things in healthcare environment using elliptic curve cryptography, *IEEE Internet of Things Journal*, 2 (1), 72–83, 2014.

[2] Moosavi, S. R., Gia, T. N., Nigussie, E., Rahmani, A. M., Virtanen, S., Tenhunen, H., and Isoaho, J. End-to-end security scheme for mobility enabled healthcare Internet of Things, *Future Generation Computer Systems*, 64, 108–124, 2016.

[3] Laplante, P. A., and Laplante, N. The internet of things in healthcare: Potential applications and challenges, *IT Professional*, 18 (3), 2–4, 2016.

[4] Blagojce, J., Ivan, K., Katarina, T., Ivika, D., and Suzana, L. Mammographic Image Classification Using Texture Features, 9th Conference for Informatics and Information Technology, 2012.

[5] Parthasarathy, P., and Vivekanandan, S. Investigation on uric acid biosensor model for enzyme layer thickness for the application of arthritis disease diagnosis, *Health Information Science Systems*, 6, 1–6, 2018.

[6] Varadharajan, R., Priyan, M. K., Panchatcharam, P., Vivekanandan, S., and Gunasekaran, M. A new approach for prediction of lung carcinoma using back propagation neural network with decision tree classifiers, *Journal of Ambient Intelligence and Humanized Computing*, 1–12, 2018.

[7] Lokesh, S., Kumar, P.M., Devi, M.R., Parthasarathy, P., and Gokulnath, C. An automatic Tamil speech recognition system by using bidirectional recurrent neural network with self-organizing map, *Neural Computing Applications*, 31 (5), 1–11, 2018.

[8] Abubacker, N. F., Azman, A., Doraisamy, S., and Murad, M. A. A. An integrated method of associative classification and neuro-fuzzy approach for effective mammographic classification, *Neural Computing Applications*, 28 (12), 3967–3980, 2017.

[9] Kumar, I., Bhadauria, H. S., Virmani, J., and Thakur, S. A hybrid hierarchical framework for classification of breast density using digitized film screen mammograms, *Multimedia Tools Applications*, 76 (18), 18789–18813, 2017.

[10] Dora, L., Agrawal, S., Panda, R., and Abraham, A. Optimal breast cancer classification using Gauss–Newton representation based algorithm, *Expert System Applications*, 85, 134–145, 2017.

[11] Abdel-Zaher, A. M., and Eldeib, A. M. Breast cancer classification using deep belief networks. *Expert System Applications*, 46, 139–144, 2016.

[12] Cong, J., Wei, B., He, Y., Yin, Y., and Zheng, Y. A selective ensemble classification method combining mammography images with ultrasound images for breast cancer diagnosis, *Computational and Mathematical Methods in Medicine*, 2017.

[13] Wang, Z., Xiao, X., Song, H., Wang, L., and Li, Q. Development of anatomically realistic numerical breast phantoms based on T1-and T2-weighted MRIs for microwave breast cancer detection, *IEEE Antennas and Wireless Propagation Letters*, 13, 1757–1760, 2014.

[14] Shankar, K., Lakshmanaprabu, S. K., Gupta, D., Maseleno, A., and De Albuquerque, V. H. C. Optimal feature-based multi-kernel SVM approach for thyroid disease classification, *Journal of Supercomputing*, 76, 1–16, 2018.

[15] Lakshmanaprabu, S. K., Mohanty, S. N., Shankar, K., Arunkumar, N., and Ramirez, G. Optimal deep learning model for classification of lung cancer on CT images, *Future Generation Computer Systems*, 92, 374–382, 2019.

[16] Shankar, K., Elhoseny, M., Lakshmanaprabu, S. K., Ilayaraja, M., Vidhyavathi, R. M., Elsoud, M. A., and Alkhambashi, M. Optimal feature level fusion based ANFIS classifier for brain MRI image classification, *Concurrency and Computation: Practice and Experience*, e4887, 1–12, 2018.

[17] Elhoseny, M., and Shankar, K. Optimal bilateral filter and convolutional neural network based denoising method of medical image measurements, *Measurement*, 143, 125–135, 2019.

[18] Shankar, K., Lakshmanaprabu, S. K., Khanna, A., Tanwar, S., Rodrigues, J. J., and Roy, N. R. Alzheimer detection using Group Grey Wolf Optimization based features with convolutional classifier, *Computers & Electrical Engineering*, 77, 230–243, 2019.

[19] Suresh, R., Rao, A. N., and Reddy, B. E., Detection and classification of normal and abnormal patterns in mammograms using deep neural network, *Concurrency and Computation: Practice and Experience*, 31 (14), e5293, 2019.

9 Artificial Intelligence with a Cloud-Based Medical Image Retrieval System Using a Deep Neural Network

9.1 INTRODUCTION

Recently, the exponential development of clinical multimedia data using the Internet of Healthcare Things (IoHT) in Hospital Information Management Systems (HIMS), and many other domains such as health data retrieval, clustering, recommendation, etc., has become applicable in several ways. The IoHT-based applications require effective models to withstand the content-based multimedia retrieving process. It has been assumed that a major application of medical images as well as management, query, and investigation play a vital role in smart HIMS [1]. Several types of medical images are produced every year, which is a massive challenge in healthcare organizations since it requires effective management and distributing data at the same time as cost reduction. Also, it is evaluated that medical imaging data storage takes up more space than other data. Several types of experiments are carried out in medical image indexing and querying in the high-dimensional data [2–4]. It intends to work in a centralized manner which does not include massive data. The query abilities are unsatisfactory due to the improved response time along with the improved size of the searching file. Hence, the deployment of maximum performing medical image query techniques is significant in future enhancements.

Here, Cloud computing has provided a gradual transition in the delivery model of information technology from a product to a service. It has enabled the availability of different software, platform and infrastructural resources as scalable services on demand through the internet. The cloud offers virtual centralization, memory, and so on, where it is used by a web-friendly device like a system, laptop, smartphones, etc. Mobile cloud (MC) is referred to as the class of reliable computing structure with a massive number of processing nodes that tend to provide reformed computing abilities for various users at any place and time. To acquire the whole energy of MC power, productive data management is the most essential one for tackling a large number of medical images as well as simultaneous end users. Also, the MC platform gives a location-based query that activates medical users to collect patient data as well as images. This can be accomplished by using a scalable, higher-throughput, position-based querying, and indexing mechanism.

The specificity of imaging methods and imaging features of clinical images are composed of major images without B-images that are named as grayscale images. Hence, color is not important to differentiate medical images. Shape features are the most required one with the desired parameter. Likewise, images with maximum similarity do not have the shape for retrieving the same symptoms. Therefore, the texture feature is more essential in medical image prediction that is based on pathology determination. Specifically, in the case of pathological analysis, the textures of normal organs and diseased parts vary, and textures mimic the spatial homogeneity of the image.

Texture features can be applied for capturing granularity as well as recurring patterns. In the case of color images and unwanted shaped images, developers have presented the image retrieval (IR) model based on multifeature integration. Wanjun et al. [3] computed the Euclidean distance of color histogram as well as the texture feature of an image, respectively. As a result, the Euclidean distances have been concatenated to obtain similarity value. Yanping et al. [4] filtered color features from hue saturation value (HSV) space and the Gray-Level Co-concurrence Matrix (GLCM) feature, whereas GLCM fused Tamura features to create a dense amount of texture features. Bing et al. [5] attained third-order color features, three texture features using Tamura, and shape features by applying Fourier that combines to form the IR technique according to multifeature combination.

Under the application of wavelet transforms as well as GLCM, features are extracted for the IR process [6]. The texture feature vectors using GLCM are calculated for every image by the use of mean and standard variance. In addition, the contrast, correlation coefficient, as well as the entropy of GLCM are also used. Following, similarity values are applied with diverse weights of Euclidean distances in the form of a reputed outcome. Zhou et al. [7] extracted texture features with the application of GLCM and Tamura from the DDSM database for the IR task. Anran et al. [8] showcased that, based on the frequency attributes of medical images, features of frequency distribution and amplitude can be attained under the investigation of medical images. Based on diverse frequency values, an IR model of spectral similarity has been presented.

Jinge [9] performed a similar process on the human brain as well as the lungs. The Tamura method was more applicable for feature extraction in human brain images using a similar function. The GLCM model is adaptable for images of the human heart. Luo et al. [10] completed image preprocessing on an insight toolkit (ITK) environment. The Tamura approach was applied for extracting texture features of segmented images as well as checked using heart computed tomography (CT) images. Gao [11] computed the iris structure intensity under the application of Tamura texture features and computed the relationship among iris fiber structure as well as desired features. Jun [12] integrated the direction of Tamura, a morphological task with Gaussian blurring, and effectively produced latitude and longitude arrangement of a distribution map.

Kumar [13] deployed an image database of eyes, with the intensity of eye images to create feature vectors, and employed Euclidean distances for retrieving eye images. Ou [14] defined, as well as obtained texture by Gabor wavelet transform for retrieving skin images. Anwar [15] applied rapid wavelet transform for extracting detailed coefficients of images. The standard deviation (SD) as well as kurtosis of images is determined, and the Euclidean distance was utilized for estimating the distance among features of query image (QI) and every image of the database. Chunyan et al. [16] aimed at the security of medical IR process, with integrated features of Henon mapping to process frequency domain cryptographic functions on an image, and degraded the encrypted image using wavelets, and a model of encrypted medical IR relying on discrete wavelets as well as perceptual hash were projected. Some other deep learning–based medical diagnosis models have also been presented in the literature [17–20].

This study presents a new deep neural network (DNN) with directional local ternary quantized extrema patterns (DLTerQEPs) and a crest line–based cloud-based medical image retrieval model called the DC-DNN model. The proposed DC-DNN model involves distinct levels such as feature extraction, similarity measurement, image retrieval, and image classification. In the earlier stage, a pair of features, namely texture and shape features, are extracted from the input image. Following, similarity measurement takes place utilizing the Euclidean distance metric. Simultaneously, the DNN-based classifier technique is employed for classifying the retrieved images. In the end, the retrieved image undergoes classification and allocates class labels for each input image.

9.2　THE PROPOSED DC-DNN MODEL

The process involved in a cloud-based image retrieval system is shown in Fig. 9.1. The training images and testing images undergo the DC-DNN process in the cloud server to retrieve the related images. The complete operation involved in the DC-DNN technique has illustrated in Fig. 9.2. From the figure, it is clear that the DLTerQEPs and Crest lines models are used as a feature extractor to derive the texture and edge features. Then, the affinity among images placed in a database and QI has been computed in the feature space with the help of the Euclidean distance value. After the images are retrieved, DNN-relied image classification is carried out.

9.2.1　DLTerQEP-Based Texture Feature Extraction

DLTerQEP explains the spatial local texture in the case of ternary patterns under the application of local extrema and dimensional geometric infrastructures. For

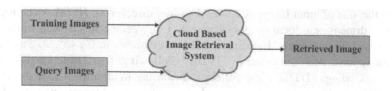

FIGURE 9.1　Cloud-based image retrieval system.

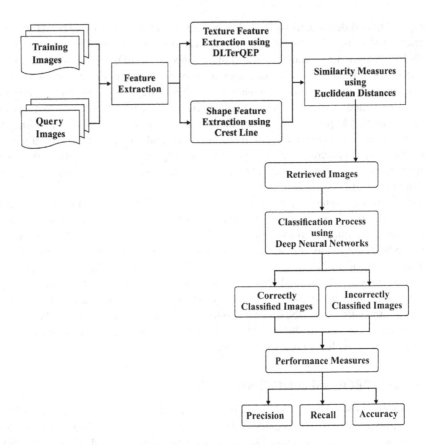

FIGURE 9.2 Overall process of proposed DC-DNN model.

DLTerQEP, local extrema in each direction are essential to computing with local differences from middle and adjacent pixels by indexing the patterns with pixel locations.

The locations undergo indexing using four directional extremum operator evaluations. Local directional extrema values (LDEV) for local pattern neighborhoods of an image (IM) are valued in Eq. (9.1)

$$LDEV(q,r) = \sum_{q=1}^{z_1}\sum_{r=1}^{z_1}\left[IM(q,r) - IM(1 + floor(z_1/2), 1 + floor(z_1/2))\right] \quad (9.1)$$

where the size of input image is $z_1 \times z_1$. The four directional, $HVDA_7$ structures of possible dimensional local quinary patterns (LQP) geometries is used in the feature extraction operation. The directional local extrema in 0°, 45°, 90°, and 135° directions have been extracted in HVDA7. Following, four Directional Ternary Extrema Codings (DTECs) are collected according to additional four directions from different thresholds under the application of the local ternary patterns (LTP) model.

9.2.2 CREST LINE–BASED SHAPE FEATURE EXTRACTION

Here, it is developed with automated crest line extraction of used medical images. It is comprised of three phases. Initially, a step that has initial curvatures and directions on all vertices of triangulation, the next step manages crest point classification, and the last step is to monitor the crest lines.

9.2.2.1 Curvature Approximation

The initial step is:
   For each vertex v_i of a mesh,

1. Obtain the star of v_i, pointed by a *star(vi)*.
2. Fix the quadratic patch (2) on v_i and *star(vi)*.
3. Determine the principal curvatures as well as the adjacent directions on v_i, as defined in the previous stage.

9.2.2.2 Crest Point Classification

In crest line, a vertex point has been identified as the crest point. The local neighborhood of vertex v of the triangulated mesh is a *star(v)*. It is applied as well as directly evaluates the directional derivative of the maximum curvature of all vertices, but the gradient is noise sensitive and does not offer the reliable measures when required, especially on irregular triangulated meshes. Finally, the given rules were applied in this method. Once the higher principal curvature k_1 and corresponding domain direction t_l on vertex v are calculated, some of the domain values of the *star(v)* are given in the following:

- The domain measures of *star(v)* are $(u_1 u_L)$, where L represents a value of vertices in *star(v)* and u_0 denotes the domain of v.
- Identify the facet that conjunction t_1 and obtain two vertices u_{m1} and u_{m2}, $m\{1, 2\} \in [1, L]$.
- Follow a similar direction - t_1 and obtain vertices u_{j1} and u_{j2}, $j\{1, 2\} \in [1, L]$.
- Obtain maximum curvatures k_1^{m1m2}, k_1^{j1j2} on points U_{m1m2} and U_{j1j2} by interpolating with (k_1^{m1}, k_1^{m2}) and (k_1^{j1}, k_1^{j2}).
- If $(k_1^0)^2 - (k_1^{m1m2})^2 > e$ and $(k_1^0)^2 - (k_1^{j1j2})^2 > e$ then v is a crest point, where $e > 0$ manages the maximality.

It has been employed to limit the arithmetic errors on the number of crest points. In addition, k_1^i implies the largest curvature on vertex $u_i, 0 \le i \le L$.

9.2.2.3 Crest Lines

The model is comprised of managing sources in crest point classification. However, it has been reached to find the crest vertices that are not applicable. Also, there is a requirement of developing technology to combine all points and deploy features of an object. It is constrained with two portions. Initially, it is observed with every crest line and, secondly, it concatenates the massive number of lines, respectively.

Suppose the mesh is comprised of N vertices. The steps are:

1. Initiate line list LS and fix several lines $j = 0$.
2. Fix the id of recent vertex $i = 0$.
3. When v_i is not visited, if a crest point contains two crest points on the star then:
   - call *traceCrestLine(vi, ls_j, (v_i, ls_j, "first")*.
   - call *traceCrestLine(vi, ls_j, (v_i, ls_j, "last")*.
   - Improve j.
4. When $i < N$, increase i and go to Step 3.

When a crest point is constrained with one or more crest points on the star and classified into a cross crest point, the start tracing line leads to the issue of the ambiguity of choosing a path. A cross crest point is named as a bifurcation point. A crest line bifurcates more than two lines. Due to the lack of advance link of a point, until tracing stop criteria and apply the latter portion of join lines.

The procedure *traceCrestLine* (vi, ls_j) is:

1. Mark v_i as visited and include it to line ls_j.
2. Obtain every vertex of *star(vi)*, which are crest points that are not visited. Suppose their number be n.
3. When $n = 1$, then go to Step 1 for novel vertex, otherwise exit.

9.2.3 EUCLIDEAN DISTANCE–BASED SIMILARITY MEASUREMENT

In the content based medical image retrieval (CBMIR) method, Euclidean distance has been used for identifying similarity from the images. The distance from two images is employed to compute the similarity between images. Euclidean distance is one of the vital distance values. It is computed with the application of the Minkowski Distance equation by fixing p's value as 2. For two diverse images x and y, it upgrades the distance d using the equation

$$d(x,y) = \sqrt{\sum_{i=1}^{n}(x_i - y_i)^2} \tag{9.2}$$

9.2.4 DNN-BASED CLASSIFICATION

The DNN basically operates on the feed-forward networks model along with the greedy layer. In this model, the data flow is initiated from the input layer to the output layer with no looping task. A major benefit of the DNN classification model is the probability of a missing value is minimum. The DNN concept implements with a single layer in the unsupervised pretraining phase. The DNN model determines a classification value $f(x)$ at the prediction time. Each input data $x = [x_1, \ldots, x_N]$ is named as forward pass. Here, f implies function that has a series of layers that is shown in Eq. (9.3)

$$Z_{ij} = x_i w_{ij}; Z_j = \sum_i Z_{ij} + b_j; X_j = g(Z_j) \qquad (9.3)$$

where input layer is denoted as x_i, output layer is x_j, w_{ij} are model parameters; and $g(Z_j)$ analyzes the mapping task. Layer-wise relevance propagation degrades the classification as output $f(x)$ with respect to relevance's r_i, which has input component x_i, which involves in the classifier decision as given in Eq. (9.4)

$$f(x) = \sum_i r_i \qquad (9.4)$$

where $r_i > 0$ is the positive classification decision and $r_i < 0$ is negative evidence; otherwise, it is referred to as neutral evidence, although the relevance attribute r_i is computed under the application Eq. (9.5). The common structure of a DNN is presented in Fig. 9.3.

$$r_i = \sum_j \frac{Z_{ij}}{\Sigma_i Z_{ij}} \qquad (9.5)$$

The DNN is capable of examining the unknown feature coherences of input. The DNN offers a hierarchical feature learning method. Hence, the higher-level features can be retrieved from minimum level features with a greedy layer–based unsupervised pretraining stage. Hence, the main goal of a DNN is to manage the complex functions that present high-level abstraction.

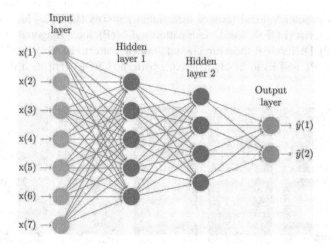

FIGURE 9.3   DNN architecture.

TABLE 9.1
Data Set Description

Description	Values
Database	NEMA CT
Number of Images	600
Image Size	512×512
Number of Classes	10
Classes Distribution	54, 70, 66, 50, 15, 60, 52, 104, 60, 69

9.3 PERFORMANCE VALIDATION

9.3.1 DATA SET USED

To ensure the proficient outcome of the projected DC-DNN model, benchmark NEMA CT images are applied for experimentation [21]. This offers accurate details of the representing capabilities to precisely differentiate the images. The details are listed in Table 9.1, and holds a total of 600 images with pixel dimensions of 512×512. Moreover, a collection of 10 classes are present in the applied data set. A few of the sample images are shown in Fig. 9.4.

9.3.2 RESULTS ANALYSIS

Fig. 9.5 depicts the visual outcome of the presented technique at the time of retrieving images. The outcome indicated that the appropriate images present in the database are effectively retrieved by the projected DC-DNN technique.

A comprehensive investigation of the simulation results takes place by the DC-DNN technique over the compared approaches concerning precision, recall, and accuracy and is illustrated in Figs. 9.6–9.8. A set of methods used for comparison purposes are local ternary directional patterns (LTDP), local quantized extrema patterns (LQEP), local mesh patterns (LMeP), local diagonal extrema pattern (LDEP), DLTerQEP, local directional gradient pattern (LDGP), local Weighting Pattern (LWP), and local block-difference pattern (LBDP). Through the precision

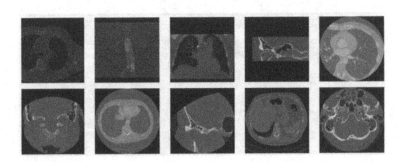

FIGURE 9.4 Sample test images.

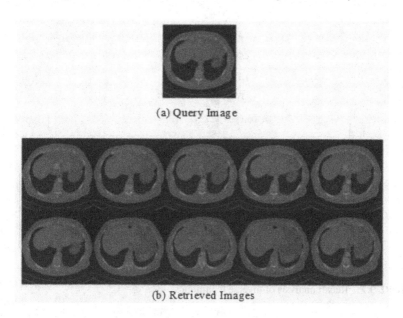

(a) Query Image

(b) Retrieved Images

FIGURE 9.5 Sample of retrieved results.

investigation of the results exhibited by the DC-DNN technique, it can be observed that the following approaches such as LTDP, LQEP, and LMeP techniques achieve minimal precision values of 8.97%, 8.93%, and 8.91% correspondingly. It is also observed that somewhat effective precision is provided by the following LDEP, DLTerQEP, and LDGP techniques with the precision values of 10.27%, 9.10%, and 10.27%. Also, the LWP and LBDP techniques exhibit acceptable precision values of

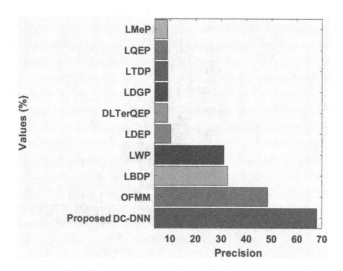

FIGURE 9.6 Precision analysis of diverse techniques.

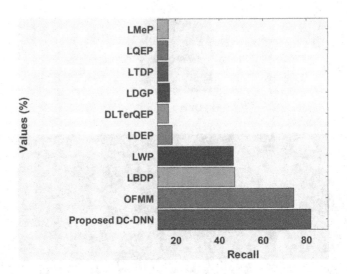

FIGURE 9.7   Recall analysis of diverse techniques.

31.03% and 32.57%. Moreover, the OFMM technique reaches the closer precision value of 48.51%. But, the DC-DNN technique leads to outstanding results by achieving the highest precision value of 80.84%.

During the assessment of the results with respect to recall, it is displayed that the following DLTerQEP, LTDP, LQEP, and LMeP techniques lead to worse classifier results with the recall values of 16.68%, 16.59%, 16.55%, and 16.66% correspondingly. Along with that, somewhat better results are achieved by the LDEP and LDGP techniques by offering near identical recall values of 18.39% and 17.28%. At the same time, the LWP and LBDP techniques have reached acceptable recall values

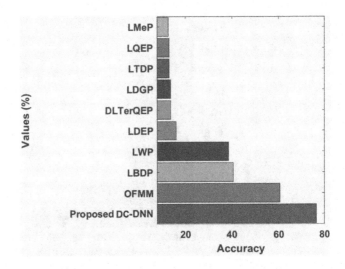

FIGURE 9.8   Accuracy analysis of diverse models.

of 46.51% and 47.11%. Just as, the OFMM technique offers near optimal classifier results with a recall value of 74.12%. But, the DC-DNN technique leads to outstanding results by achieving the highest precision value of 81.94%.

While assessing the outcome of the presented DC-DNN technique in terms of accuracy, it is verified that LTDP, LQEP, and LMeP techniques offer the lowest accuracy values of 12.94%, 12.85%, and 12.64% correspondingly. After that, a little higher accuracy values are exhibited by the LDEP, DLTerQEP, and LDGP techniques with the accuracy of 15.96%, 13.62%, and 13.51%. Along with that, the LWP and LBDP techniques demonstrate moderate and closer accuracy values of 38.54% and 40.61%. Concurrently, the OFMM technique offers a near maximum accuracy value of 60.52%. But, the DC-DNN technique leads to outstanding results by achieving the highest accuracy value of 76.40%. By mentioning the above stated results, it is provided that the DC-DNN technique has offered ultimate retrieval and classification performance under several dimensions.

9.4 CONCLUSION

This study has introduced an effective cloud-based DC-DNN model to proficiently retrieve medical images. The proposed DC-DNN model involves four main processes, namely feature extraction, similarity measurement, image retrieval, and image classification. The feature extraction process makes use of two techniques to retrieve the shape and texture features. Besides, similarity measurement takes place using Euclidean distance followed by DNN-based classification. For testing, a set of test images from NEMA CT image data set is applied. The attained simulation results ensured that the DC-DNN model has resulted in effective retrieval and classification performance by attaining maximum precision of 67.98%, a recall of 81.94% and an accuracy of 76.40%. As a part of future work, the secure retrieval of images can be carried out by the use of cryptographic algorithms.

REFERENCES

[1] Ansari, S., Aslam, T., Poncela, J., Otero, P., and Ansari, A., Internet of Things-based healthcare applications, in *IoT Architectures, Models, and Platforms for Smart City Applications*, IGI Global, 2020, 1–2.
[2] Qadri, Y. A., Nauman, A., Zikria, Y. B., Vasilakos, A. V., and Kim, S.W. The future of healthcare Internet of Things: A survey of emerging technologies, *IEEE Communications Surveys & Tutorials*, 22 (2), 1121–1167, 2020.
[3] Wanjun, L., and Hongwei, Z. Image retrieval of improved color and texture features based on wavelet transform, *Computer Engineering and Applications*, 52 (17), 181–186, 2016.
[4] Yanping, G., Hongbing, G., and Zhiying, R. Image retrieval algorithm combining color feature and texture feature, *Wireless Internet Technology*, 2017.
[5] Bing, L. On technology of computer image retrieval based on multi feature fusion, *Journal of Southwest China Normal University (Natural Science)*, 42 (1), 54–59, 2017.
[6] AoBo, Z., Xianbin, W., and Zhang, X. Retrieval algorithm for texture image based on improved dual tree complex wavelet transform and gray gradient co-occurrence matrix, *Computer Science*, 44 (6), 274–277, 2017.

[7] Zhou, J., Feng, C., Liu, X., and Tang, J. A texture features based medical image retrieval system for breast cancer, in *Proceedings of the International Conference on Computing Convergence Technology*, 8562, 1010–1015, 2013.

[8] Anran, M., Ning-ning, R., Li-bo, H., Yong, S., Shao, Y., and Jian-feng, Q. Image retrieval based on medical digital X-ray spectrum characteristics, *Chinese Journal of Medical Physics*, 33 (9), 933–938, 2016.

[9] Jinge, G. *The Research and application of medical image retrieval technology based on texture feature*, Inner Mongolia University of Science Technology, 2012.

[10] Luo, R., Rui, L., Liu, R. G., Ye, C., and Guan, Z. Z. Total knee arthroplasty for the treatment of knee osteoarthritis caused by endemic skeletal fluorosis, *Chinese Journal of Tissue Engineering Research*, 16, 1555–1557, 2012.

[11] Gao, Y., Song, H., and Zhang, Z. J. Calculation method of iris structure density based on Tamura features, *Computer Technology & Development*, 26 (3), 36–39, 2016.

[12] Jun, M., Senlin, Z., and Zhen, F. Recognition algorithm of fabric based on Tamura texture features, *Light Industry Machinery*, 35 (4), 2017.

[13] Kumar, M. Content based medical image retrieval using texture and intensity for eye images, *International Journal of Scientific & Engineering Research*, 7 (9), 2016.

[14] Ou, X., Pan, W., Zhang, X., and Xiao, P. Skin image retrieval using Gabor wavelet texture feature, *International Journal of Cosmetic Science*, 38 (6), 607–614, 2016.

[15] Anwar, S. M., Arshad, F., and Majid, M. Fast wavelet based image characterization for content based medical image retrieval, in *Proceedings of the 2017 International Conference on Communication, Computing and Digital Systems, C-CODE 2017*, Pakistan, March 2017, 351–356.

[16] Chunyan, Z., Jingbing, L., and Shuangshuang, W. Encrypted image retrieval algorithm based on discrete wavelet transform and perceptual hash, *Journal of Computer Applications*, 38 (2), 539–544, 2018.

[17] Elhoseny, M., Bian, G. B., Lakshmanaprabu, S. K., Shankar, K., Singh, A. K., and Wu, W. Effective features to classify ovarian cancer data in internet of medical things, *Computer Networks*, 159, 147–156, 2019.

[18] Kathiresan, S., Sait, A. R. W., Gupta, D., Lakshmanaprabu, S. K., Khanna, A., and Pandey, H. M. Automated detection and classification of fundus diabetic retinopathy images using synergic deep learning model, *Pattern Recognition Letters*, Vol. 159, 2020.

[19] Shankar, K., Perumal, E., and Vidhyavathi, R. M. Deep neural network with moth search optimization algorithm based detection and classification of diabetic retinopathy images. *SN Applied Sciences*, 2 (4), 1–10, 2020.

[20] Raj, R. J. S., Shobana, S. J., Pustokhina, I. V., Pustokhin, D. A., Gupta, D., and Shankar, K. Optimal feature selection-based medical image classification using deep learning model in Internet of Medical Things, *IEEE Access*, 8, 58006–58017.S, 2020.

[21] Murala, S., Wu, Q. M. J. MRI and CT image indexing and retrieval using local mesh peak valley edge patterns, Signal Process, *Image Communication*, 29 400–440, 2014.

10 IoHT with Cloud-Based Brain Tumor Detection Using Particle Swarm Optimization with Support Vector Machine

10.1 INTRODUCTION

Rapid development in data and micro-electromechanical system (MEMS) methods results in the deployment of the Internet of Things (IoT), which enables objects, data, and virtual environments to interact with each other [1]. Various fields apply IoT in data collection tasks such as transport, homes, hospitals, cities, etc. The exponential development of IoT-dependent healthcare tools and sensors exist in real time [2]. With an increased cost of medications as well as the existence of diverse diseases all over the world, it is significant for healthcare from a hospital-based structure to a patient-centric structure. To control the disease, the ubiquitous sensing capabilities derived from IoT devices were applied to detect the possibilities of developing the disease for a user. The interconnection of IoT and CC is assumed to be more applicable in monitoring affected people in remote areas by providing enough support for physicians [3]. IoT has been provisioned by the application of virtual unconstrained utilities as well as resources of cloud computing (CC) to maintain technical shortcomings such as storage, processing, and power. Simultaneously, CC provides the merits of IoT under the expansion of its value to deal with real-time applications and to provide massive facilities in a distributed as well as dynamic fashion. Therefore, IoT and CC could be applied for developing novel applications and services in the healthcare domain [4].

IoHT is an alternate combination of IoT and healthcare, which has been deployed in the healthcare sector [5]. In the case of massive IoT domains, the major duty of big data analytics as well as CC is a popular methodology. Ma et al. [6] proposed a backend structure that activates cognitive facilities in healthcare recommending that a cloud approach must not be basically homogeneous and offers medical data transfer and CC service layers. The BT affects people at all age groups and it results in increased death rate [7]. A tumor is comprised with tissues of anomalous or abnormal cells. Also, it is associated with a benign BT, which is noncancerous and does not spread to neighboring tissues; however, it is malicious and can cause death.

An alternate case named malignant BTs is referred to as cancerous, which is developed in the brain and uniquely breeds when compared with benign tumors and spreads in nearby tissues. Magnetic resonance imaging (MRI) has been applied to gain knowledge of tumors and calculate the spreading value. T1-weighted and T2-weighted scans are MRI scan types that are applied. To point to tissue regions that are alleviated in T1 scans, water and fat molecules are differentiated. Losses of tissues are represented by darker areas. Under the insertion of nonradioactive unit gadolinium, the infected visibility could be enhanced with additional inflammatory lesions. An extraordinary water content tissue is more visible as hyperintense points in T2 scans, which present tissue loss regions.

Cerebrospinal fluid (CSF), white matter (WM), and gray matter (GM) are assumed to be diverse tissues that are present in the brain. Intensity, position, textural features, and tumor structures are more specific whereas MRI brain images develop the segmentation complex. However, it is not sufficient and wavelet features, gray-level-based features, local binary patterns (LBPs), and the Gray-Level Co-occurrence Matrix (GLCM) could be obtained. There is no requirement of labeling; independent tumor segmentation is processed by doctors in disease diagnosis. Among other patients, glioblastoma multiforme (GBM) BTs are commonly detected tumors in the brain. Due to the structure, texture, and shape difference, robotic tumor segmentation is more crucial, which tends to result in false positive, soft tissues, and blood vessels, which are assumed to be nontumor brain structures that are nonidentified as tumors. Various types of conventional models perform completely independent tumor segmentation. Hence, tumor identification is a classical segmentation technique that is manual and not completely automatic.

A numerous sum of brain MRI scans is essential to deploy classifiers like machine learning (ML) for BT segmentation with the ground truth of different real-time applications for training. In developing the optimal classification model, factors are assumed to have classification accuracy, algorithm functions, as well as processing resources [8]. With the application of methods like unsupervised classification, such as FCM and Self Organizing Map (SOM), and supervised approaches, such as k-nearest neighbor (K-NN), SVM, and artificial neural network (ANN), the brain MRI is classified. Generative, as well as discriminative approaches, are two types of automated segmentation of BT.

For comparison with independent methods, Menze et al.'s [9] previous work represents that models are based on discriminative classification that indicates optimal function. The association between the ground truth as well as input image is known by discriminative models based on feature extraction [10]. With respect to ground truth, the value is valuable and applies the methods of supervised learning in several cases, which acquires a higher data set. To attain the unknown tumor segments, advanced profit in healthy tissues is used. Hence, it is a complex operation to transform previous knowledge into proper probabilistic techniques.

Soft computing models like fuzzy entropy values are used in selecting the best features. GLCM is assumed to be a statistically relied feature extraction method. GLCM distributes the pixel measures in case of identical gray-level values. In the comparison of classification models, the back propagation neural network (BPNN) model has maximum prediction accuracy value. The learning model investigates the application of predefined data to attain training data for extracting Harlick texture features from every MRI [11]. The attained results from existing models reveal that the Elman Network with log sigmoidal activation function is adaptable when compared with alternate ANNs with higher performance value. Under the application of ANN classification, the grades of tumors are computed with a maximum accuracy [12]. The above task applies an automatic prediction as well as the segmentation model. Following, a median filter has been utilized for eliminating gray as well as white noise. The BT analysis is forecasted using fast bounding box (FBB) schemes.

The ANN employs features to train data with the help of pretrained data and performs the tumor classification. It applies a grading matrix of Grade (II–IV) of three grades. The histogram is employed to estimate the intensity of 2D images. Also, the obtained histogram signal has been used to Slantlet transform to perform the feature extraction process [5]. Binary classification model is operated according to NN, the system undergoes training under the application of pretrained feature data, and it has been classified automatically using an Alzheimer's disease pathological brain. Also, various conventional models are used in tumor segmentation. Thus, to identify the tumors, the classical segmentation is manually not accurate. Few works make use of different AI techniques to diagnose the disease effectively [13–17].

This chapter devises an effective IoHT with CC-based BT identification model by the use of GLCM and PSO with SVM. The proposed PSO-SVM-based detection model comprises preprocessing, feature extraction, and classification. After completing the preprocessing stage, the feature vectors will be extracted from the preprocessed image. Finally, the PSO-SVM classifier model is applied for the classification of BT images as benign or malign. The presented GLCM-PSO-SVM model is validated using a set of images from the brain tumor segmentation (BRATS) data set. The simulation outcome ensured that the GLCM-PSO-SVM model is effective in terms of sensitivity, accuracy, and specificity.

10.2 THE PROPOSED GLCM-PSO-SVM MODEL

The block diagram of the developed GLCM-PSO-SVM system is applicable in predicting tumors in MRI as depicted in Fig. 10.1. In this model, an individual is forecasted completely by exploiting medical tools with IoT gadgets. After capturing the MRI brain images, it can be preprocessed. Hence, the features were extracted from the preprocessed image. Class labeling is more applicable to train the model. If a method is trained exactly, the testing process is initialized when images are classified in corresponding labels. The trained model is capable of testing the provided MRI brain images effectively.

10.2.1 PREPROCESSING

Brain MRI is subjected to corruption by noise while processing image transmission as well as digitization as shown in Fig. 10.2. Preprocessing is operated to eliminate the noises from MRI. The extracranial tissues such as bone, skin, and hair are rejected and result in the conversion of heterogeneous images to homogeneous images. Noise can be eliminated with the application of filters and even corrupted

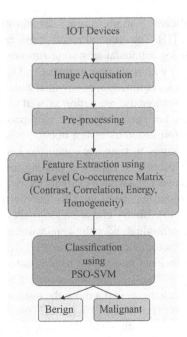

FIGURE 10.1 Working process of the GLCM-PSO-SVM model.

with minimum data of an image. Additionally, traditional filters make a smoother image constantly and develop stronger edges of an image.

It is applied with an anisotropic diffusion filter to preprocess the brain MRI since the filter avoids the noise and saves the edges. In the case of a corrupted image, the features are blurred. Here, it is employed with anisotropic diffusion filtering for denoising. The filter ranges the neighboring pixels on the basis of intensity, and a median value can be computed for pixels after estimation. A novel median value has been replaced using a central pixel.

10.2.2 FEATURE EXTRACTION

The GLCM is a model matrix utilized to determine the texture design with modeling texture as the 2D array gray-level difference. These attributes exist between a

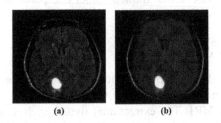

FIGURE 10.2 Preprocessing output (a) input image, (b) preprocessed image.

group of features to determine the pixel contrast as well as the power of ROI. This feature is more useful for separating the normal tissue from anomalous tissue based on removed contrast and power. It is assumed to be the statistical approach that considers spatial connection between the pixels, because it is a gray-level spatial dependence matrix. The GLCM facet is computed in four directions: 0°, 45°, 90°, and 135°; and for four distances: 1, 2, 3, and 4. Also, there are four characteristics in the GLCM (contrast, energy, homogeneity, and correlation) and can be estimated with the given functions

$$Contrast = \sum \left(|i-j|^2 \times p(i,j) \right) \tag{10.1}$$

$$Energy = \sum p(i,j)^2 \tag{10.2}$$

$$Homogeneity = \frac{\sum p(i,j)}{1+|i-j|} \tag{10.3}$$

$$Correlation = \sum (i-\mu i)(j-\mu j)\frac{p(i,j)}{[\sigma i \cdot \sigma j]} \tag{10.4}$$

The number of gray levels used in computing is the GLCM size. A matrix unit $P(i,j | \Delta x, \Delta y)$ is said to be a relative frequency, and somewhere two pixels are separated with pixel distance $(\Delta x, \Delta y)$ in the provided region, with intensity i and intensity j.

The GLCM $P[i,j]$ is comprised of a location of pixels by related gray level and referred to as identifying displacement vector $d = (dx, dy)$ and calculates each pair of pixels that has been partitioned using d that is comprised of gray levels of i and j. Wavelet is determined as a mathematical function signifying tiny waves that are scaled, as well as shifted models called a mother wavelet

$$\Psi_{a,b} = \frac{1}{\sqrt{a}} \Psi\left(\frac{t-b}{a}\right) \tag{10.5}$$

where a implies a scaling variable and b denotes as a shifting parameter. The wavelet transform (WT) considers the image on different resolution scales and changes the image to a multiresolution image through various frequency modules. The wavelet is said to be discontinuous and refers to a step function. For a function f, the Haar WT is determined as

$$f \rightarrow \left(a^L | d^L\right) \tag{10.6}$$

where L represents the disintegration level, a signifies the approximation sub-band, and d mimics the extended sub-band. The WT has been implemented to each row and column of the image accomplished from the previous level. The final has been classified as four sub-bands: LL, HL, LH, and, where L = Low, H = High. An estimation of actual image is added in the LL sub-band, while alternate sub-bands are constrained with missing rates. The LL sub-band can be attained at diverse stages that have been degraded as LL, HL, LH, and HH sub-bands. Law's energy texture features states that initially, 1D kernels of brain image are reformed to 2D filter kernels. The second step has filtering of input mammogram images under the application of Law's 2D kernels and processes the energy of an image.

10.2.3   PSO-SVM-Based Classification

10.2.3.1   SVM Classifier

The SVM is constrained with maximum accuracy, simple mathematical tractability, geometrical representation, and so on. Thus, solutions attained are unique and global to eliminate the convergence of local minimum executed under the application of alternate types of statistical learning methods such as NN. It is offered with a p-dimensional training data set of N size with respect to

$$\{(x_n, y_n) \mid x_n \in R^p, y_n \in \{-1, +1\}\}, n = 1, \ldots, N \tag{10.7}$$

where y_n is $a - 1$ or 1 by means of class 1 or 2. Each x_n is said to be a p-dimensional vector. A maximum-margin hyperplane, which segments class 1 from class 2, is highly applicable in SVM. Hence, a type of hyperplane is described as

$$wx - b = 0 \tag{10.8}$$

where w implies a normal vector of hyperplane and b signifies the bias. It highly concentrates on selecting w and b to improve the margin among two parallel hyperplanes of higher size while isolating the data. Therefore, two parallel hyperplanes are expressed using the given equation

$$wx - b = \pm 1 \tag{10.9}$$

This model could be converted into an optimizing problem. The purpose of this technique is to boost the distance of two parallel hyperplanes and remove the data falling from the margin. Under the application of elegant mathematical data, this issue can be resulted in

$$\min \| w \| \tag{10.10}$$

$$s.t. \; y_n(wx_n - b) \geq 1, n = 1, \ldots, N.$$

Practically, $\| w \|$ is replaced by applying

$$\min \frac{1}{2} \| w \|^2 \tag{10.11}$$

$$s.t. \; y_n(wx_n - b) \geq 1, n = 1, \ldots, N.$$

The major reason depends upon the function of $\| w \|$, which is relevant in calculating the square root value. Once the value has been computed, the solution cannot be changed, and modify the problems as optimizing quadratic programming, which becomes simpler by applying Lagrange multipliers and reputed quadratic programming techniques. It undergoes mapping of binary classification issues, expressed as

$$\min \frac{1}{2} \| w \|^2 + C \sum_{n=1}^{N} \xi_n \tag{10.12}$$

where C is a regularizing variable and ξ_n represents the penalizing relaxation parameter.

10.2.3.2 Parameter Optimization of SVM Using the PSO Algorithm

For validating the optimal parameter of C, the trial-and-error method is implemented. Therefore, implementation of these techniques tends to overhead in action without any assurance of attaining optimized outcomes. It is the application of PSO that is employed for uniquely optimizing parameters. It is linked by global optimization, accomplished from learning fish training or bird flocking. Then, the cross-validation (CV) model is deployed to invent the fitness function (FF) that is applied in PSO. It encloses a swarm of particles that is extended for all iterations. To attain an optimized result, every particle updates its best position (p_{best}) and best global position in swarm (g_{best}) as defined below

$$p_{best_i} = p_i\left(k^*\right) \tag{10.13}$$

$$s.t.\, \text{fitness}(p_i(k^*)) = \min, [\text{fitness}(p_i(k))],$$

$$g_{best} = p_{i^*}(k^*) \tag{10.14}$$

$$s.t.\, \text{fitness}(p_{i^*}(k^*)) = k = i \min, [\text{fitness}(p_i(k))],$$

where i is the particle index, P implies the overall particles, k denotes the iteration index, z shows the recent iteration value, and p represents the position. The velocity as well as position of particles is improved using the provided functions

$$v_i(z+1) = wv_i(z) + c_1 r_1\left(p_{best_i}(z) - p_i(z)\right) + c_2 r_2\left(g_{best}(z) - p_i(z)\right) \tag{10.15}$$

$$p_i(z+1) = p_i(z) + v_i(z+1) \tag{10.16}$$

where v is velocity. The inertia weight w is applied to manage the global searching as well as a local application. The r_1 and r_2 are distributed in a uniform model by random variables in a range $(0, 1)$. The c_1 and c_2 are positive constant variables named as acceleration coefficients. Thus, the particle undergoes encoding as embedded by parameters C.

10.3   EXPERIMENTAL ANALYSIS

10.3.1   DATA SET DESCRIPTION

The verification of the projected GLCM-PSO-SVM method is carried out by applying standard open access data set BRATS 2015, which is comprised of a collection of MRI images [18]. The execution portion is implemented by the MATLAB tool with 1.70 GHz GPU Processor and 6 GB internal RAM. The applied data set is composed of three different brain MRI image sub data sets such as Training, Leader Board, and Challenge, as shown in Fig. 10.3.

Here, it is applied with the Training and Challenge data set. It is comprised of high-grade tumor (HGT) images and low-grade tumor (LGT) images with ground truth images from different radiologists. The MRI images of the training data set

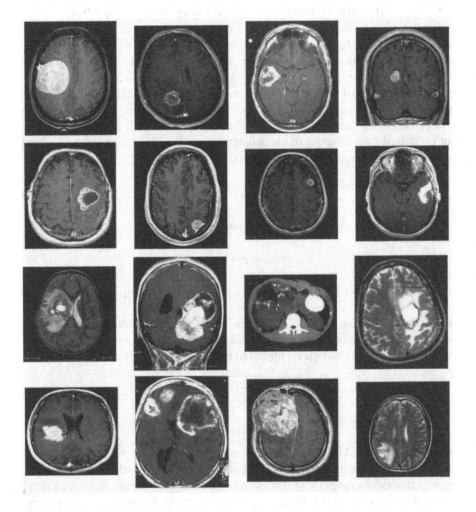

FIGURE 10.3   Sample images.

have been used in classification training of the proposed scheme. Therefore, access can be made via online to calculate the outcome of provided techniques. The data set has images of two types: benign and malignant.

10.3.2 EVALUATION METRICS

To examine the outcome of the GLCM+PSO-SVM approach, a comparative investigation is processed among output images with ground truth images. According to the expert's knowledge, the ground truth images are produced. An exactly classified nontumor image has been presented as true positive (TP) and an accurately classified tumor image is expressed as true negative (TN). Hence, the incorrectly classified tumor image is given as false positive (FP) and the incorrectly classified nontumor image is presented as false negative (FN). Such variables are computed according to the comparison with ground truth images.

A collection of values applied in estimating the function as given below ranges from 0 and 100. The values applied are

$$\text{Sensitivity} = \frac{TP}{TP + FN} \tag{10.16}$$

$$\text{Specificity} = \frac{TN}{TN + FP} \tag{10.17}$$

$$\text{Accuracy} = \frac{TP + TN}{TP + FN + TN + FP} \tag{10.18}$$

10.3.3 RESULTS ANALYSIS

Table 10.1 provides a relative examination of projected and existing models on the classification of BT images. Fig. 10.4 examines the results analysis of distinct techniques [19] in terms of sensitivity. The method developed by Anitha et al. (2017) demonstrated its ineffective outcome with a minimum sensitivity value of 91.20%. Next, the technique developed by Urban et al. (2014) exhibited a slightly higher sensitivity value of 92.60%. Afterward, the methods devised by Pereira et al. (2016) and

TABLE 10.1
Comparisons of Proposed with State of the Arts Methods

Methods	Sensitivity	Specificity	Accuracy
GLCM+PSO-SVM	97.08	96.12	97.96
Selvapandian et al. (2018)	96.20	95.10	96.40
Anitha et al. (2017)	91.20	93.40	93.30
Pereira et al. (2016)	94.20	94.40	94.60
Urban et al. (2014)	92.60	93.00	93.30
Islam et al. (2013)	94.30	95.10	95.90

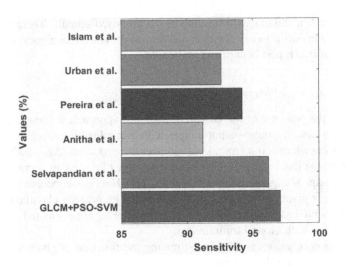

FIGURE 10.4 Sensitivity analysis of distinct models.

Islam et al. (2013) have resulted in a moderate and near-identical sensitivity value of 94.20% and 94.30%, respectively. The model introduced by Selvapandian et al. (2018) has shown compete results by offering a near-optimal sensitivity value of 96.20%. However, the GLCM-PSO-SVM model has reached a maximum sensitivity of 91.20%.

Fig. 10.5 investigates the analysis of the results of distinct techniques with respect to specificity. The method coined by Urban et al. (2017) depicted its ineffective result with a minimum specificity value of 93.00%. Next, the technique developed by Anitha et al. (2017) exhibited a slightly higher specificity value of 93.40%. Later,

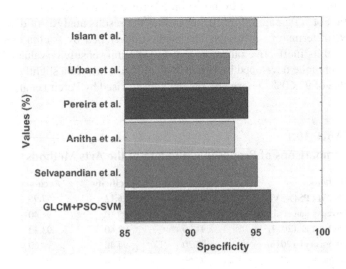

FIGURE 10.5 Specificity analysis of distinct models.

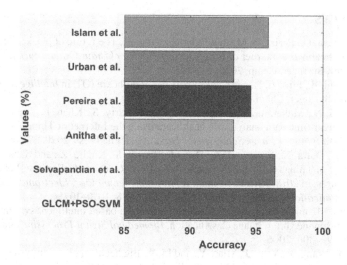

FIGURE 10.6 Accuracy analysis of distinct models.

the methods devised by Pereira et al. (2016) resulted in moderate and near-identical specificity values of 94.40%. The model developed by Selvapandian et al. (2018) and Islam et al. (2013) has shown compete results by offering a near optimal specificity value of 95.10%. Therefore, the GLCM-PSO-SVM systems has reached a maximum specificity of 96.12%.

Fig. 10.6 forecasts the results analysis of distinct techniques by means of accuracy. The technique deployed by Anitha et al. (2017) demonstrated its ineffective outcome with a minimum accuracy value of 93.30%. Next, the technique developed by Urban et al. (2014) exhibited a slightly higher accuracy value of 93.30%. Then, the methods devised by Pereira et al. (2016) and Islam et al. (2013) have resulted in moderate and near identical accuracy values of 94.60% and 95.90%, correspondingly. The model introduced by Selvapandian et al. (2018) has shown compete results by offering a near-optimal accuracy value of 96.40%. But, the GLCM-PSO-SVM model has reached a maximum accuracy of 97.96%.

10.4 CONCLUSION

This chapter has introduced a proficient GLCM-PSO-SVM model to identify and classify BTs with the use of IoHT and CC. The projected model operates on three stages: preprocessing, feature extraction, and classification. GLCM-based feature extraction and PSO-SVM-based image classification processes are carried out. The presented PSO-SVM model is validated using a set of images from the BRATS data set. The simulation outcome ensured that the PSO-SVM model is effective in terms of sensitivity, accuracy, and specificity. The experimental outcome ensured that the GLCM-PSO-SVM model has reached maximum classifier results with the highest sensitivity of 97.08%, a specificity of 96.12% and an accuracy of 97.96%. As part of future work, the presented technique results could be improvised by the use of segmentation approaches.

REFERENCES

[1] Srivastava, G., Parizi, R. M., and Dehghantanha, A., The future of blockchain technology in healthcare internet of things security, in *Blockchain Cybersecurity, Trust and Privacy*, Springer, Cham, 2020, 161–184.

[2] Farahani, B., Firouzi, F., and Chakrabarty, K., Healthcare IOT, in *Intelligent Internet of Things* Springer, Cham, 2020, 515–545.

[3] Sahu, S. N., Moharana, M., Prusti, P. C., Chakrabarty, S., Khan, F., and Pattanayak, S. K., Real-time data analytics in healthcare using the Internet of Thing, in *Real-Time Data Analytics for Large Scale Sensor Data*, Academic Press, 2020, 37–50.

[4] Paul, P., Dutta, N., Biswas, B. A., Das, M., Biswas, S., Khalid, Z., and Saha, H. N. An Internet of Things (IoT) Based System to Analyze Real-time Collapsing Probability of Structures, in *2018 IEEE 9th Annual Information Technology, Electronics and Mobile Communication Conference (IEMCON)*, IEEE, 2018, 1070–1075.

[5] Maitra, M., and Chatterjee, A. A Slantlet transform based intelligent system for magnetic resonance brain image classification, *Biomedical Signal Processing and Control*, 1 (4), 299–306, 2006.

[6] Ma, Y., Wang, Y., Yang, J., Miao, Y., and Li, W. Big health application system based on health internet of things and big data, *IEEE Access*, 5, 7885–7897, 2017.

[7] Abbasi, S., and Tajeripour, F. Detection of brain tumor in 3D MRI images using local binary patterns and histogram orientation gradient, *Neurocomputing*, 219, 526–535, 2017.

[8] El-Dahshan, E.S.A., Mohsen, H.M., Revett, K., and Salem, A.B.M. Computer-aided diagnosis of human brain tumor through MRI: A survey and a new algorithm, *Expert Systems with Applications*, 41 (11), 5526–5545, 2014.

[9] Menze, B., Reyes, M., Jakab, A., Gerstner, E., Kirby, J., Kalpathy-Cramer, J., and Farahani, K., NCI-MICCAI challenge on multimodal brain tumor segmentation, in Proceedings of NCI-MICCAI BRATS, Nagoya, Japan, 2013.

[10] Geremia, E., Zikic, D., Clatz, O., Menze, B. H., Glocker, B., Konukoglu, E., Shotton, J., Thomas, O. M., Price, S. J., Das, T., and Jena, R., Classification forests for semantic segmentation of brain lesions in multi-channel MRI, in *Decision Forests for Computer Vision and Medical Image Analysis*, Springer, London, 2013, 245–260.

[11] Hussein, E., and Mahmoud, D. Brain tumor detection using artificial neural networks, *Journal of Science Technology*, 13, 31–39, 2012. http://www.sustech.edu/staff publications/20130323072020220.pdf.

[12] Sharma, Y. and Chhabra, M. An Improved Automatic Brain Tumor Detection System. *International Journal of Advanced Research in Computer Science and Software Engineering*, 5 (4), 11–15, 2015.

[13] Shankar, K., Elhoseny, M., Lakshmanaprabu, S. K., Ilayaraja, M., Vidhyavathi, R. M., Elsoud, M. A., and Alkhambashi, M. Optimal feature level fusion based ANFIS classifier for brain MRI image classification, *Concurrency and Computation: Practice and Experience*, 32 (1), 1–12, 2018.

[14] Elhoseny, M., and Shankar, K. Optimal bilateral filter and convolutional neural network based denoising method of medical image measurements. *Measurement*, 143, 125–135, 2019.

[15] Shankar, K., Lakshmanaprabu, S. K., Khanna, A., Tanwar, S., Rodrigues, J. J., and Roy, N. R. Alzheimer detection using Group Grey Wolf Optimization based features with convolutional classifier, *Computers & Electrical Engineering*, 77, 230–243, 2019.

[16] Elhoseny, M., Shankar, K., and Uthayakumar, J. Intelligent diagnostic prediction and classification system for chronic kidney disease, *Scientific Reports*, 9 (1), 1–14, 2019.

[17] Lakshmanaprabu, S. K., Mohanty, S. N., Krishnamoorthy, S., Uthayakumar, J., and Shankar, K. Online clinical decision support system using optimal deep neural networks, *Applied Soft Computing*, 81, 105487, 2019.

[18] MRBrainS18, Grand Challenge on MR Brain Segmentation at MICCAI, 2018, available at https://mrbrains18.isi.uu.nl/

[19] Selvapandian, A., and Manivannan, K. Fusion based glioma brain tumor detection and segmentation using ANFIS classification, *Computer Methods and Programs in Biomedicine*, 166, 33–38, 2018.

11 Artificial Intelligence-Based Hough Transform with an Adaptive Neuro-Fuzzy Inference System for a Diabetic Retinopathy Classification Model

11.1 INTRODUCTION

The influence of the Internet of Health Things (IoT) on the progression of the healthcare industry is enormous and the utilization of artificial intelligence (AI) has transformed IoHT systems at almost every level. In general, diabetic retinopathy (DR) occurs in people who have been suffering from diabetes for a long period and, due to retinal infection, this leads to loss of eyesight. With the application of these models of fundus imaging, the DR-defected retinal structure can be predicted. The fundus images are captured with the application of a fundus camera. The inner surface of the eye is shown by fundus images that are composed with fovea, retina, blood vessels, optic disc (OD), as well as macula. An ordinary retina is composed of blood vessels that are constrained with nutrients and blood supply. The blood vessels are soft and filled with extra blood pressure, and may burst in diabetic patients. By providing additional small blood vessels count, the DR develops owing to the extra pressure exist at the retinal surface. To classify the different stages of DR such as non-proliferative DR(NPDR) and proliferative diabetic retinopathy (PDR) over actual retina, the blood vessels development can be applied as the bio-marker [1].

More developers have been presented with efficient vessel segmentation over the last few decades and retinal images undergo classification based on the disease severity [2, 3]. In the case of DR analysis, an automatic retinopathy classifier has been deployed based on artificial neural networks (ANNs). Genetic algorithm (GA) and fuzzy c-means (FCM) can be applied to attain maximum accuracy value [4]. These models are multilayered thresholding [5] in segmenting blood vessels present in DR images. The retinal structure investigation deals with ridgelet [6], curvelet [7] and wavelet [8] transforms that are utilized with fundus images. Fuzzy logic (FL) is employed to provide higher sensitivity value. With the application of a multiscale line detecting device, the retinal vascular can be analyzed [9]. The combination of a Gaussian mixer and nearest neighborhood approaches is employed in [10], who deployed a scheme named DR analysis by applying machine learning (DREAM) and processed the classification task by using support vector machine (SVM). An L2 Lebesgue integral model was applied to compute the infinite perimeter regularization [11]. To preprocess the image, the global thresholding approach has been employed [12]. The blood vessel prediction by morphological component analysis (MCA) reached maximum accuracy value [13].

The technique of deep neural networks (DNNs) [14] has been used, which undergoes training across a greater number of sample STARE, CHEST, and DRIVE data sets. However, it has a manageable number of samples. For system-based screening, a telemedicine system has been deployed by utilizing red lesions of retinopathic images. In the case of DR referral [15], a direct technology is presented by classification training. The reduction of lesion-to-lesion prediction requires numerous pools to perform the classifier training. Many traditional methods such as morphological gradients, wavelets, NN, and alternate computation have to be executed to provide efficient and accurate DR prediction at earlier phases. However, these techniques are more tedious to be computed.

Automatic DR detection techniques are composed with various benefits such as DR can be forecasted at primary stages in an effective manner. Some of the methodologies such as deep learning (DL) have led to the evolution of computer vision. The image classification task is performed by convolution neural networks (CNNs). Research of this application contributes in feature segmentation as well as blood vessels [16]. The actual image classification can be processed by the application of deep CNNs (DCNNs) by classifying DR fundus images. To resolve the issues involved in segmentation of blood vessel, a CNN method is employed in [17] to retrieve image features. Therefore, it is comprised with few limitations of existing methodologies. Then, data sets that have minimum quality and lower fundus images with individual collection platform provide few difficulties for comparing the model's function. In order to enhance the working function of a method, AlexNet is devised.

Additionally, the qualified models of CNNs are GoogleNet and VGGNet. Recently, the projected Residual Network (ResNet) is assumed to be a more vital system that increments the CNNs function at the time of processing image classification. To increase the learning duration and compare with traditional approaches namely, VGGNet, AlexNet, and GoogleNet, it is employed with transfer learning that provides exact as well as automated prediction with visual infections to be lowered at the minimum degree [5, 18]. Among other models, the presented approaches are composed with consecutive improvements on convergence time for a huge-sized data set and shows qualified function rather than classification.

In this chapter, it is deployed with the automatic segmentation–centric classification method for DR. At this point, contrast-limited adaptive histogram equalization (CLAHE) has been employed for preprocessing and the watershed technique is used in image segmentation. Then, the Hough transform (HT)–based feature extraction process is carried out by the adaptive neuro-fuzzy inference system (ANFIS) method utilized in image classification. In experimental analysis, the data set has been derived from the Kaggle website, which is assumed to be an open-source environment that tries to develop the DR detecting approach.

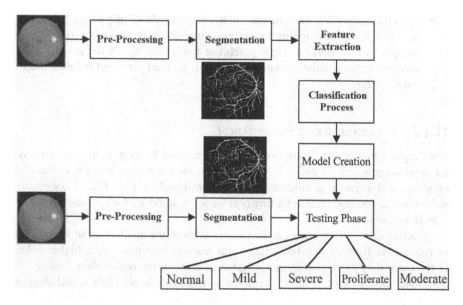

FIGURE 11.1 Overall process of the presented model.

11.2 PROPOSED METHOD

The entire computation of the projected segmentation centric classifier is depicted in Fig. 11.1. The input image is preprocessed. Later, the preprocessed image is induced to a watershed-based segmentation task. The CLAHE technique is employed in segmentation operation. Following, the HT-based feature extraction is carried out by the ANFIS classifier that has been developed using the appropriate training stage. After the deployment of these models, test input images are given to reach the exact result.

11.2.1 PREPROCESSING

In case of local areas, to eliminate the extra noise, the enhancement is limited in CLAHE. A massive number of valid histograms intensity could be evaluated using CLAHE. These approaches are based on the exclusive image area and distribute the histogram to avoid extra amplification, as well as intensity values, and undergo remapping under the application of shared histograms. Some of steps in the CLAHE mechanism are provided as follows:

- Derive whole inputs: Number of areas in row and columns, count of bins for histograms used in developing image transformation, clip limit to reduce contrast from 0 to 1.
- Process each contextual area to develop mappings: Derive individual image and deploy a region histogram under the application of finite bin count, clip the histogram by exploiting clip limit, and produce mapping for this region.

- For collecting a CLAHE image, interpolate gray-level mappings: Extract the cluster of four mapping functions, compute image area of overlapping mapping tiles, obtain a single pixel, use four mappings of the pixel, and interpolate the simulation outcome to attain the final pixel and reiterate the entire image.

11.2.2 WATERSHED-BASED SEGMENTATION

The height value of the landscape can be monitored by gray values of particular pixel magnitudes. In every local minimum, the catchment basin is composed of steepest descent at a minimum as demonstrated in Fig. 11.2. Concerning noisy clinical images, numerous tiny regions were deployed for segmentation and feature extraction.

Effective feature extraction can be performed with the application of voxel-wise morphometric features that have maximum features comprised of a higher value of the same data and noise as the presence of error in the registration strategy. A traditional model for reaching the regional features is to apply prior knowledge, in which a permanent region of interest (ROI) has a voxel-wise feature. However, it is not efficient during the application of various forms to reflect images, because ROI features from alternate templates.

Let $I_i^j(v)$ is a voxel-wise cell thickness rate at voxel u in kth template of ith training subject, $i \in [1, N]$. The ROI portion depends upon concatenated discrimination as well as robust measure, $DRM^j(v)$, resulting from N training subjects of feature importance as well as spatial reliability.

$$DRM^j(v) = P^j(v)C^j(v) \qquad (11.1)$$

where P^j refers to the Pearson correlation (PC), and $C^j(v)$ shows the spatial steadiness from other features of spatial neighborhood. Watershed segmentation has been computed on each DRM^j map to reach the ROI. The Gaussian kernel has been employed to smooth every map DRM^j to eliminate additional segmentation. Finally, the kth template has been divided as overall R^j nonoverlapping areas; which has been pointed out that each template provides a result from the ROI region.

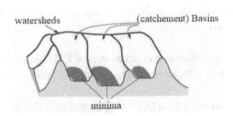

FIGURE 11.2 Concept of watershed transform.

11.2.3 HOUGH TRANSFORM–BASED FEATURE EXTRACTION

This approach is more vital image-processing models that are applied in segmenting features of a specific inside an image. The transform among Cartesian space as well as parameter space has been described by a straight line. The main aim of this approach is to identify ineffective samples from specific classes by the histogram voting procedure. It is considered as parameter space, of object variants as local maxima termed as accumulator space, which has been deployed by the model to compute the HT.

The local maxima have been employed in the training of back propagation neural networks (BPNNs). The HT could be arithmetically presented for lines, circle, or ellipse. It is mainly employed to discover lines from images; however, it is differed for identifying alternate shapes. For instance, (x, y) is a point of the binary image. In method $y = ax + b$, every pair of (a, b) are allocated into accumulator array. When $(x, y) = (1, 1)$, the function relevant a and b is $1 = a$, $1 + b$, and expressed as $b = -a + 1$. Therefore, the line $b = -a + 1$, is comprised of each pair of points to a single point $(1, 1)$ as illustrated in Fig. 11.3.

11.2.4 ANFIS-BASED CLASSIFICATION

The infrastructure of ANFIS is comprised of seven inputs as well as a single output. The seven inputs show the diverse textural features estimated from every image. All training sets create a fuzzy inference system with 16 fuzzy rules. Every input has been provided with two generalized bell curve membership function (MF) and results were indicated by two linear MF. The simulation outcome of 49 rules is condensed into 1 output, showing the system result for desired input images. A classification design of the ANFIS utilizes both ANN and FL. The ANFIS classification forms if–then principles and combine input and output learning techniques. It is utilized to train the ANFIS classification. For instance, the ANFIS classification contains seven inputs $(x_1, x_2, x_3, x_4, x_5, x_6, x_7)$ and one outcome (y). A first-order Sugeno fuzzy method with base fuzzy if–then rules are represented as Eq. (11.2). If $x_1 A_1$ and $x_2 B_1$ and $x_3 C_1$ and $x_4 D_1$ and $x_5 E_1$ and $x_6 F_1$ and $x_7 G_1$ then

$$f_1 = px_1 + ppx_2 + qx_3 + qqx_4 + sx_5 + ssx_6 + rx_7 + u \qquad (11.2)$$

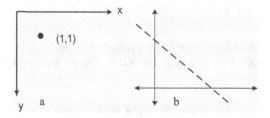

FIGURE 11.3 (a) point in an image and its corresponding line in transform for an image and (b) transform.

where p, pp, q, qq, s, ss, r, and u are linear outcome parameters. A design of ANFIS classification is designed utilizing 5 layers and 256 if–then rules:

Layer-1: All node i is a square node through the node function.

$$O_{1,i} = \mu_{A_i}(x_1), \; for \; i = 1,2,$$

$$O_{1,i} = \mu_{B_i}(x_2), \; for \; i = 3,4,$$

$$O_{1,i} = \mu_{C_i}(x_3), \; for \; i = 5,6,$$

$$O_{1,i} = \mu_{D_i}(x_4), \; for \; i = 7,8,$$

$$O_{1,i} = \mu_{E_i}(x_5), \; for \; i = 9,10,$$

$$O_{1,i} = \mu_{F_i}(x_6), \; for \; i = 11,12,$$

$$O_{1,i} = \mu_{G_i}(x_7), \; for \; i = 13,14, \tag{11.3}$$

where $x_1, x_2, x_3, x_4, x_5, x_6$, and x_7 are inputs to node i and A_i, B_i, C_i, D_i, E_i, F_i, and G_i are linguistic labels connected by node function. However, $O_{1,i}$ is the membership function of A_i, B_i, C_i, D_i, E_i, F_i, and G_i. Generally, $\mu_{A_i}(x_1)$, $\mu_{B_i}(x_2)$, $\mu_{C_i}(x_3)$, $\mu_{D_i}(x_4)$, $\mu_{E_i}(x_5)$, $\mu_{F_i}(x_6)$, and $\mu_{G_i}(x_7)$ are selected to bell-shape by maxima equivalent to 1 and minima equivalent to 0, namely

$$\mu_i(x_i) = \exp((-(x_i - c_i)/(a_i))^2) \tag{11.4}$$

where a_i, c_i denote the parameter sets. A parameter can be presented as premise parameters.

Layer-2: All nodes are circle node labeled Π that improves the incoming signals and forwards product. For example

$$O_{2,i} = w_i$$

$$= \mu_{A_i}(x_1) \cdot \mu_{B_i}(x_2) \cdot \mu_{C_i}(x_3) \cdot \mu_{D_i}(x_4) \cdot \mu_{E_i}(x_5) \cdot \mu_{F_i}(x_6) \cdot \mu_{G_i}(x_7)$$

$$i = 1,2,3,\ldots,256. \tag{11.5}$$

Every node outcome indicates the firing strength of a rule.

Layer-3: All nodes are circle node labeled N. The ith node computes the ratio of each rule:

$$O_{3,i} = \bar{w}_i = \bar{w}_i / (w_1 + w_2 + \cdots + w_{256}),$$

$$i = 1,2,3,\ldots,256. \tag{11.6}$$

Layer-4: All nodes i is a square node by node function

$$O_{4,i} = \bar{w}_i \cdot f_i$$

$$= w_i \cdot (px_1 + ppx_2 + qx_3 + qqx_4 + sx_5 + ssx_6 + rx_7 + u)$$

$$i = 1, 2, 3, \ldots, 256. \tag{11.7}$$

where w_i is the resultant of layer 3, and $\{p_i, pp_i, q_i, qq_i, s_i, ss_i, r_i, u_i\}$ is a parameter set. The parameters are presented as a subsequent vector.

Layer-5: A single node is circle node labeled $\sum$ that calculates the entire result as the outline of every input signal:

$$O_{5,i} = overall\ output = \sum_i \bar{w}_i f_i = \frac{\sum_i w_i f_i}{\sum_i w_i} \tag{11.8}$$

11.3 PERFORMANCE ANALYSIS

11.3.1 DATA SET DESCRIPTION

To estimate the efficient segmentation and DR classification, it is applied with the HT-ANFIS technique as proposed and processed with other previous models under the application fundus image data set. The data set has been retrieved from the Kaggle [19] website that is an open source that tries to develop DR prediction method.

The eye images of high-definition are composed of a data set and graded by trained experts into five categories as given in Table 11.1. Fig. 11.4 depicts the improvement of DR from the robust retina to PDR. The data set is comprised of red green blue (RGB) images that have resolution up to 35,126 with 3500 × 3000 resolution. The labels are provided by experts where they are ranked as DR presence by a scale 0, 1, 2, 3, 4, that is derived from normal, mild, moderate, severe, and proliferative.

11.3.2 RESULTS ANALYSIS

Fig. 11.5 illustrates the segmentation outcome of the HT-ANFIS of the DR image data set. It is shown that the HT-ANFIS effectively segments the input images.

TABLE 11.1

Data Set Description

Class Name	DR Grades	No. of Images
Class 0	Normal	25810
Class 1	Mild	2443
Class 2	Moderate	5291
Class 3	Severe	873
Class 4	Proliferative	708

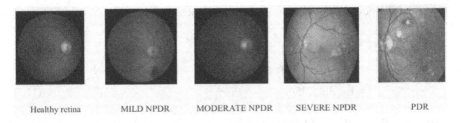

Healthy retina   MILD NPDR   MODERATE NPDR   SEVERE NPDR   PDR

FIGURE 11.4   Stages of DR starting from a healthy fundus image.

A comparison of the results offered by the HT-ANFIS has been made with respect to diverse measures. Fig. 11.6 investigates the accuracy analysis of diverse models on the applied DR data set. On measuring the classifier results in terms of accuracy, an ineffective DR classifier result has been demonstrated by the VGGNet-16 model with an accuracy value of 48.13%. Along with the previous value, it is exhibited that the VGGNet-s model has resulted in a slightly higher accuracy value of 73.66%. Simultaneously, it is indicated that the VGGNet-19 has attained an even higher accuracy value of 82.17%. Concurrently, it is noticed that the ResNet model leads to a moderate classifier outcome with an accuracy of 90.40%. Besides, a competitive accuracy value of 93.36% has been achieved by the GoogleNet model whereas the HT-ANFIS model showcases effective results with a maximum accuracy of 94.65%.

Fig. 11.7 examines the sensitivity analysis of various methods on the applied DR data set. On measuring the classifier results by means of sensitivity, ineffective DR classifier results have been shown by the VGGNet-s model with a sensitivity of 33.43%. In the same way, it is exhibited that the VGGNet-19 model has resulted in a slightly higher sensitivity value of 54.51%. At the same time, it is indicated that the GoogleNet model has attained an even higher sensitivity value of 77.66%.

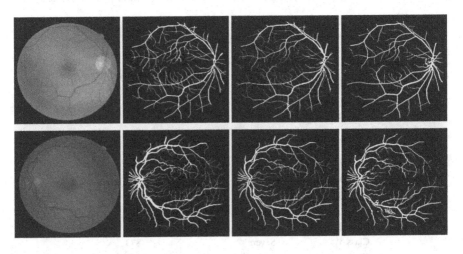

FIGURE 11.5   Segmentation results.

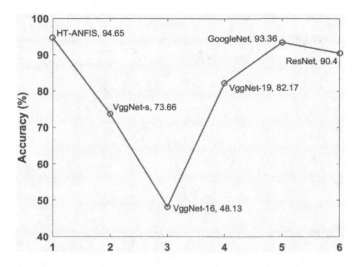

FIGURE 11.6 Comparison of classifier outcome with respect to accuracy.

Concurrently, it is noticed that the HT-ANFIS model leads to a moderate classifier outcome with a sensitivity of 80.18%. On the other hand, a competitive sensitivity value of 86.37% has been achieved by the VGGNet-16 model, whereas the ResNet model showcases effective results with a maximum sensitivity of 88.78%.

Fig. 11.8 predicts the specificity analysis of different approaches on the applied DR data set. On measuring the classifier results in terms of specificity, ineffective DR classifier results have been indicated by the VGGNet-16 model with the specificity of 29.09%. Similarly, it is shown that the GoogleNet model has resulted in a slightly better specificity value of 93.45%. Concurrently, it is pointed that the VGGNet-s model

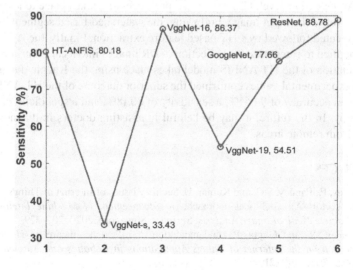

FIGURE 11.7 Comparison of classifier outcome with respect to sensitivity.

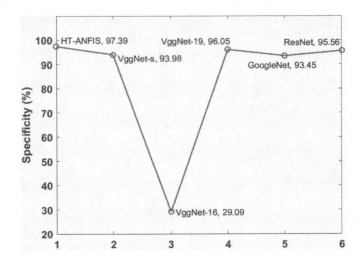

FIGURE 11.8   Comparison of classifier outcome with respect to specificity.

has accomplished an even higher specificity value of 93.98%. Simultaneously, it is clear that the ResNet model leads to a moderate classifier outcome with a specificity of 95.56%. Besides, a competitive specificity value of 96.05% has been achieved by the VGGNet-19 model whereas the HT-ANFIS model depicts efficient results with a maximum specificity of 97.39%.

11.4   CONCLUSION

This chapter has presented a completely automatic segmentation-based classification method for DR and the proposed HT-ANFIS model has performed a series of processes. At the earlier level, CLAHE-based preprocessing takes place to improve the contrast level of the input image. Following, the watershed-based segmentation process is executed followed by a HT-based feature extraction. Finally, the ANFIS classifier is applied to categorize the collection of DR images into its appropriate classes. The simulation of the HT-ANFIS model takes place using the Kaggle data set. The attained experimental values confirmed the superior outcome of the HT-ANFIS system with an accuracy of 94.65%, a sensitivity of 80.18%, and a specificity of 97.39% respectively. In the future, it may be helpful in assisting doctors in diagnosing DR patients from remote areas.

REFERENCES

[1] Pandey, P., Pandey, S.C. and Kumar, U. Security issues of Internet of Things in healthcare sector: An analytical approach, in *Advancement of Machine Intelligence in Interactive Medical Image Analysis*, Springer, Singapore, 2020, 307–329.
[2] Mahajan, R. and Gupta, P. Implementation of IoT in healthcare, in *Handbook of Research on the Internet of Things Applications in Robotics and Automation*, IGI Global, 2020, 190–212.

[3] Kathiresan, S., Sait, A. R. W., Gupta, D., Lakshmanaprabu, S. K., Khanna, A., and Pandey, H. M. Automated detection and classification of fundus diabetic retinopathy images using synergic deep learning model, *Pattern Recognition Letters*, 133, 210–216, 2020.

[4] Shankar, K., Perumal, E., and Vidhyavathi, R. M. Deep neural network with moth search optimization algorithm based detection and classification of diabetic retinopathy images, *SN Applied Sciences*, 2 (4), 1–10, 2020.

[5] Akram, M. U., and Khan, S. A. Multilayered thresholding-based blood vessel segmentation for screening of diabetic retinopathy, *Engineering Computing*, 29, 165–173, 2013.

[6] Bankhead, P., Scholfield, C. N., McGeown, J. G., and Curtis, T. M. Fast retinal vessel detection and measurement using wavelets and edge location refinement, *PLOS One*, 7 (3), 1–12, Mar. 2012.

[7] Staal, J., Abramoff, M. D., Niemeijer, M., Viergever, M. A., and Ginneken, B. v. Ridge-based vessel segmentation in color images of the retina, *IEEE Transactions of Medical Imaging*, 23 (4), 501–509, Apr. 2004.

[8] Miri, M. S., and Mahloojifar, A. Retinal image analysis using curvelet transform and multistructure elements morphology by reconstruction, *IEEE Transactions of Biomedical Engineering*, 58 (5), 1183–1192, May 2011.

[9] Nguyen, U. T. V., Bhuiyan, A., Park, L. A. F., and Ramamohanarao, K. An effective retinal blood vessel segmentation method using multiscale line detection, *Pattern Recognition*, 46, 703–715, 2013.

[10] Roychowdhury, S., Koozekanani, D. D., and Parhi, K. K. DREAM: Diabetic retinopathy analysis using machine learning, *IEEE Journal of Biomedical Health Information*, 18 (5), 1717–1728, Sep. 2014.

[11] Zhao, Y., Rada, L., Chen, K., Harding, S. P., and Zheng, Y. Automated vessel segmentation using infinite perimeter active contour model with hybrid region information with application to retinal images, *IEEE Transactions Medical Imaging*, 34 (9), 1797–1807, Sep. 2015.

[12] Mapayi, T., Viriri, S., and Tapamo, J-R. Comparative study of retinal vessel segmentation based on global thresholding techniques, *Computing and Mathematical Methods in Medicine*, 2015, 1–15, Nov. 2014.

[13] Imani, E., Javidi, M., and Pourreza, H-R. Improvement of retinal blood vessel detection using morphological component analysis, *Computer Methods and Programs in Biomedicine*, 118, 263–279, 2015.

[14] Lakshmanaprabu, S. K., Mohanty, S. N., Krishnamoorthy, S., Uthayakumar, J., and Shankar, K. Online clinical decision support system using optimal deep neural networks, *Applied Soft Computing*, 81, 105487, 2019.

[15] Pires, R., Avila, S., Jelinek, H. F., Wainer, J., Valle, E., and Rocha, A. Beyond lesion-based diabetic retinopathy: a direct approach for retinal, *IEEE Journal of Biomedical Health Information*, 21 (1), 193–200, Jan. 2017.

[16] Wang, Z., and Yang, J. Diabetic retinopathy detection via deep convolutional networks for discriminative localization and visual explanation, *arXiv preprint*, arXiv:170310757, 2017.

[17] Wang, S., Yin, Y., Cao, G., Wei, B., Zheng, Y., and Yang, G. Hierarchical retinal blood vessel segmentation based on feature and ensemble learning, *Neurocomputing*, 149, 708–717, 2015.

[18] Elhoseny, M., Shankar, K., and Uthayakumar, J. Intelligent Diagnostic Prediction and Classification System for Chronic Kidney Disease, *Scientific Reports*, 9(1), 1–14, 2019.

[19] Diabetic Retinopathy Detection dataset, available at https://www.kaggle.com/c/diabetic-retinopathy-detection/data

12 An IoHT–Based Intelligent Skin Lesion Detection and Classification Model in Dermoscopic Images

12.1 INTRODUCTION

Advanced developments of the Internet of Health Things (IoHT) have significantly changed the healthcare sector. The IoHT devices are found to be useful in the medical field of developing, testing, and trials, and they are used in hospitals and homes. Recently, skin cancer has been considered a common disease all over the world. There are different types of cancers such as melanoma, basal cell carcinoma, squamous cell carcinoma, intraepithelial carcinoma, etc. The human skin is comprised of three cells: dermis, epidermis, and hypodermis. Initially, the epidermis contains melanocytes that produce imbalanced values. For instance, melanin is generated when there is ultraviolet (UV) exposure from the sun for a long period. Anomalous growth of melanocytes tends to lead to melanoma, which is a dangerous skin cancer [3]. Based on the study of the American Cancer Society, a greater number of new cases of melanoma are occurring, which increases the mortality rate [4]. Melanoma is said to be a malignant type of cancer that leads to maximum death when compared with other types of cancer [5]. Earlier prediction of cancer is more significant and tends to increase the lifespan of an individual [6]. Therefore, finding similarities between benign and malignant lesions is a more difficult process while detecting melanoma. It is difficult to identify melanoma with the human eye, even for medical experts.

To resolve these limitations, a novel model was introduced called dermoscopy. It belongs to a noninvasive imaging technique that allows viewing the skin surface under the application of immersion fluid as well as light maximizing tools [7]. In general, it is used in the image approach in dermatology that is comprised of the improved capability of examining cancerous disease [8, 9]. Therefore, forecasting melanoma with the naked eye might provide an inaccurate and confusing solution because it depends upon the experience of dermatologists [10]. A specialized physician with no experience can examine the melanoma and offer a gradual result [8]. To overcome these limitations in detecting melanoma, computer-aided diagnosis (CAD) schemes are essential for effective analysis. There are four stages in the CAD system to discover a skin lesion: preprocessing, segmentation, feature extraction, and classification. For accomplishing a productive outcome while detecting melanoma, lesion segmentation is assumed to be the fundamental process in CAD. Hence, the segmentation task is a problematic stage due to the existence of a wider difference in texture, color, location, and lesion size, which is derived from dermoscopic images. On the other hand, the poor contrast of the image eliminates the variations of corresponding cells. Also, few artifacts such as bubbles, hair, ebony frames, ruler marks, blood vessels, and color illumination lead to a complex lesion segmentation task.

Lesion images are more significant for the classification of melanoma. Proper classification can be processed when segmentation is properly done on the cells. Segmentation of lesions of normal tissue and attaining a greater number of features are few objectives to achieving an effective diagnosis [11]. Diverse methods are presented to perform automated lesion segmentation. It is comprised of five types. Histogram threshold has been employed to explore the threshold rates to segment lesion from normal cells. Unsupervised clustering approaches are used in color space of red green blue (RGB) dermoscopic images to attain a similar region.

Edge-based, as well as region-based models, are assumed to be the edge devices and different methods are used in separating lesions. Active contour techniques are used with meta-heuristic models, genetic algorithms (GA), snake algorithms, and so forth. The last approach is termed as supervised segmentation. Here, skin lesion has been segmented with the application of decision trees (DTs), support vector machines (SVMs), and artificial neural networks (ANNs) [12]. Detailed knowledge regarding these frameworks can be reached from recent reviews of segmentation tasks that are used in skin lesions. Each technique applies minimum features that depend upon pixel features. Therefore, traditional segmentation approaches are unable to reach the desired decision as well as demerits such as fuzzy lesion boundaries, hair artifacts, low contrast, and other artifacts that cannot be analyzed. Some other automated disease diagnosis models are also available in the literature [13–16].

This chapter proposes a novel and effective pipeline for skin lesion segmentation in dermoscopic images. The scale-invariant feature transform-support vector machine (SIFT-SVM) operates using a set of subprocesses namely preprocessing, SIFT-based feature extraction, K-means clustering–based segmentation, and support vector machine-based classification. The validation of the SIFT-SVM takes place using a skin image data set and the obtained outcome pointed out the effectiveness of the applied model over the compared methods.

12.2   THE SIFT-SVM

The overall operating principle of the SIFT-SVM is shown in Fig. 12.1. In the beginning level, preprocessing takes place to enhance the input image quality. Then, the image undergoes segmentation process by the use of the K-means clustering technique. Followed by, SIFT based feature extraction takes place, which extracts the needed features from the segmented image. At last, the SVM model is applied to classify the set of images into appropriate classes.

12.2.1   BILATERAL FILTERING–BASED PREPROCESSING

Bilateral filtering (BF) is accepted as a preprocessing play to extract the noise that occurs in the dermoscopic images. Usually, the occurrence of noise leads to

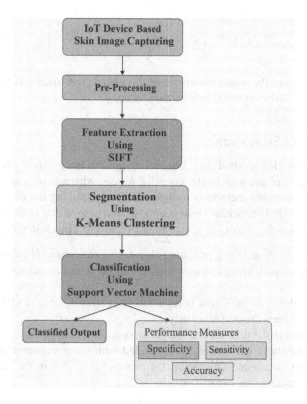

FIGURE 12.1   Block diagram of SIFT-SVM.

inefficient classifiers of the images. It can also be supposed for discriminating the noise that occurs in the initial image to the classifier. The possibility of BF is relied on a particular weight of connecting pixels to remove the noise. The simplest method for signifying a BF has the distance-based domain filter part (p, p'), and a gray-value depending on range filter part $r [(fp), (fp')]$:

$$\tilde{f}(p) = \frac{1}{N(u)} \int_{-\infty}^{\infty} f(p') d(p,p') r\big(f(p), f(p')\big) dp' \tag{12.1}$$

Where p and p' indicates the place of the intermittent and neighboring pixels, and $N(p)$ is a normalized factor.

Regarding the local mean of the neighboring pixels, the range filter part implements the value-based module to remove the noise around the boundaries. The field and range filter areas, usually a Gaussian function, is utilized and depends on the Euclidean pixel distance as denoted as

$$d(p,p') \propto \exp\left(-\frac{(p-p')^2}{2\sigma_d^2}\right) \tag{12.2}$$

$$r\big(f(u), f(u')\big) \propto exp\left(-\frac{\big(f(u) - f(u')\big)^2}{2\sigma_f^2}\right) \tag{12.3}$$

where σ_d indicates the width parameter of the filter kernel and σ_f is the noise standard deviation of the regarded regenerated value.

12.2.2 IMAGE SEGMENTATION

It can be a clustering method that classifies or clusters the group of objects in terms of the attributes or features to the count of K sets, where K indicates the positive integer. The clustering method is transferred by minimizing the distance between the information and particular cluster centroid. A distance that is utilized here is L^2 distance and is defined as $\left(d(u, v) = \sum_p (u_p - v_p)^2\right)$. The clustering play aims to cluster the information in that matching objects in a cluster and objects of dissimilar clusters are not equal. The procedure involved in the K-means method is listed here.

1. Setting the value of K that is regarded as centroids, i.e., the virtual points that have been created randomly.
2. All points in the data set are shared to its nearest centroid.
3. The position of the centroid is upgraded with the assignment of the data points to the cluster. Otherwise, the centroid is shifted to the center of its shared points.

The steps 2-3 are repeated until no centroids are moved to the subsequent round. In addition, the process gets terminated when the shift goes beyond a threshold value. The K-means method is then defining K groups of data that minimizes the subsequent objective function

$$F = \sum_{p=1}^{K} \sum_{u_q \in S_p} (u_q - c_p)^t (u_q - c_p), \tag{12.4}$$

where there exists K clusters S_p, $p = 1, 2, ..., K$, and c_i is the centroid or mean point of each point, $u_q \in S_p$. It is very useful in computer vision areas to segment the images. Each pixel that occurs in the image is connected to color as determined in RGB. The input image that requires to be segmented is defined utilizing a group of points from 3D data space. For a grayscale image, the method is equal, except that the illustration of images occurs as the gathered of points in a 1D space.

12.2.3 FEATURE EXTRACTION

This section looks at a SIFT-based feature extraction concept for extracting and explaining the feature points that require to be robust to scaling, orientation, and alteration in illumination. The group of four methods contained in the SIFT technique are:

1. Detect scale-space extrema
2. Localize feature points
3. Assignment of orientation
4. Feature point descriptor

12.2.3.1 Detect Scale-Space Extrema

Primarily, an exploring method occurs over the scale with the utilization of a Difference of Gaussian (DoG) application to search important interest points that are invariant for scaling as well as rotation. Now, scaling space is expressed as the function $L(u, v, \sigma)$ that is generated from the convolution of a variable-scale Gaussian $G(u, v, \sigma)$ containing an input image $IMG(u,v)$:

$$L(u, v, \sigma) = G(u, v, \sigma) * IMG(u, v) \tag{12.5}$$

$$G(u, v, \sigma) = \frac{1}{2\pi\sigma^2} e^{-\frac{u^2+v^2}{2\sigma^2}} \tag{12.6}$$

For efficient detection of stable key-point locations from scale space with a function of scale-space extrema in the histogram of oriented gradients (HOG) function through the image, $D(u, v, \sigma)$ is defined from the difference of two closer scales that undergo division with constant factor k:

$$D(u, v, \sigma) = (G(u, v, k\sigma) - G(u, v, \sigma)) * IMG(u,v) = L(u, v, k\sigma) - L(u, v, \sigma) \tag{12.7}$$

12.2.3.2 Localized Feature Points

A position and scaling of all interested points is calculated based on stability values that have been estimated with feature points. It is used to improve the contrast level of the images which causes the unclear image boundaries.

12.2.3.3 Assignment of Orientation

A multiple orientation has been chosen for every feature point location that depends upon the local image of gradient directions. For each image sample of $L(u, v)$, the gradient magnitude $m(u, v)$ and orientation $\theta(u,v)$ are predefined with the utilization of different pixel values

$$m(u, v) = \sqrt{\left(L(u+1,v) - L(u-1,v)\right)^2 + \left(L(u,v+1) - L(u,v-1)\right)^2} \tag{12.8}$$

$$\theta(u,v) = \tan^{-1}\left(\frac{\left(L(u,v+1) - L(u,v-1)\right)}{\left(L(u+1,v) - L(u-1,v)\right)}\right) \tag{12.9}$$

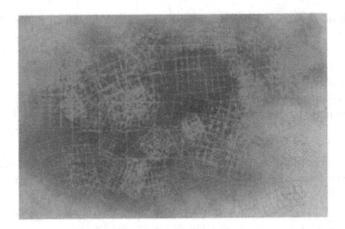

FIGURE 12.2　SIFT descriptors in a skin lesion image.

12.2.3.4　Feature Point Descriptor

A feature descriptor is an approach which considers an image and offers feature vectors. The feature descriptors encode interesting details into a sequence of numbers and plays as an arrangement of numerical "fingerprint" that can be used to differentiate one feature from another. Fig. 12.2 depicts the SIFT descriptors in a skin lesion image.

12.2.4　IMAGE CLASSIFICATION

The SVM is a type of ML method based upon the models of statistics. It can be a supervised learning method executed to identify designs in various fields. After the set of discriminate features has been selected with the earlier methods, the classification is executed to classify the various kinds of skin lesions. SVM is a supervised learning model employed for data testing, model reorganization, classifier, and regression testing. The SVM trained method generates the model that shares a novel instance through related class. In SVM, the linear function is employed so that the instances of the distinct class are separated by a clear gap. Given a train set of instance pairs (l_p, m_p), $p = 1, \cdots, n$, where $l_p \in R^n$ and $m \in \{1, -1\}^n$, the SVM requires the result of the following optimization problem:

$$\min_{w,b,\xi} \frac{1}{2} w^Z w + C \sum_{p=1}^{n} \xi_p \tag{12.10}$$

$$subject to \, m_p \left(w^Z \phi(l_p) + b \right) \geq 1 - \xi_p$$

$$\xi_p \geq 0,$$

where training vectors l_p are mapped into the highest dimensional space through the function ϕ.

Algorithm: SVM model
```
Input: T raining Image Features, Testing Image Features.
Assign: δ=resemblance among every sample that exists in the
attribute.
Output: Classified Image.
Begin
Step 1: Give data set to the model
Step 2: Features and attributes undergo classification
concerning labeled class
Step 3: Candidate Support Value evaluation
Step 4: While (Instance_value! =NULL)
Step5: Reiterate the process for every instance
Step 6: If (Support_value==δ)
Step 7: Compute Total Error Value
Step 8: End If
Step 9: If (Instance<0)
Step 10: Determine the Decision value = Support Value/Total
Error
Step 11: Reiterate the processes till empty
Step 12: End If
End
```

An SVM determines a linear separating hyperplane with maximal margin in this maximum dimensional space. $C > 0$ is the punishment attribute of the fault term. Likewise, $K(1_p, l_q) \equiv \phi(l_p)^Z \phi(l_q)$ is called the kernel function. It uses the usually implemented Radial Basis Function (RBF) determined as

$$K\left(1_p, l_q\right) = \exp\left(-\gamma \|1_p, -l_q\|^2\right), \gamma > 0 \tag{12.11}$$

In the testing procedure, the input test image is segmented and the hair extraction method occurs. Next, features are removed from the image, and the following classifier method is carried out where the input images are classification into various classes.

12.3   PERFORMANCE VALIDATION

An extensive set of simulation analysis takes place for investigating the goodness of the projected SIFT-SVM model. The results are examined under diverse dimensions, which are discussed below.

12.3.1   DATA SET USED

To validate the results of the projected SIFT-SVM model, a benchmark skin lesion data set is employed. The information related to the data set is listed out in Table 12.1 and a few test images are demonstrated in Fig. 12.3.

TABLE 12.1
Data Set Description

S. No	Classes	Number of Images
1	Angioma	21
2	Nevus	46
3	Lentigo NOS	41
4	Solar Lentigo	68
5	Melanoma	51
6	Seborrheic Keratosis	54
7	Basal Cell Carcinoma	37

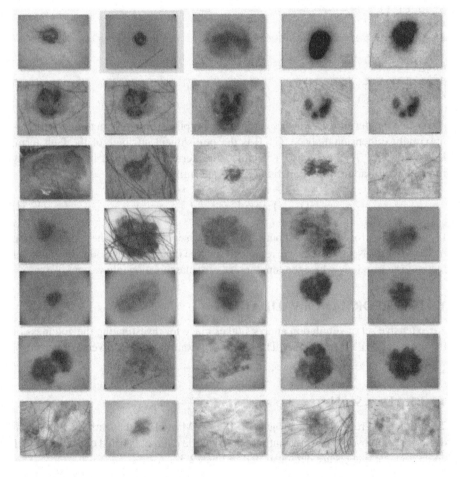

FIGURE 12.3 Sample Test Images.

12.3.2 RESULTS ANALYSIS

A clear representation of the results attained by the SIFT-SVM model is shown in Fig. 12.4. The sensitivity analysis of the SIFT-SVM with compared models is shown in Fig. 12.5. The values in Table 12.2 indicate that the Li et al. method has offered the least classifier results by offering the least sensitivity value of 82%. Then, the Yuan et al. model has provided slightly better classifier results by offering

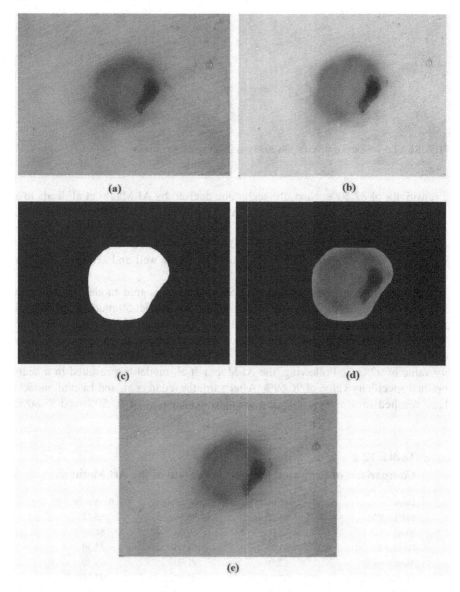

FIGURE 12.4   (a) Original image, (b) preprocessed image, (c) masked image, (d) segmented image, (e) classified image.

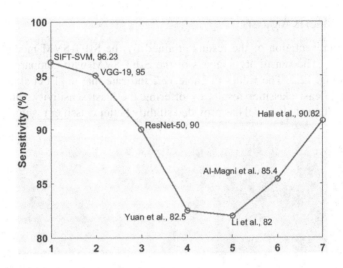

FIGURE 12.5   Comparative results analysis in terms of sensitivity.

a sensitivity of 82.50%. Next, the technique devised by Al-Magni et al. leads to a moderate sensitivity value of 85.40%. Afterward, the ResNet-50 and Halil et al. models have resulted in manageable and near-identical results of 90% and 90.82% respectively. Following, the VGG-19 model has resulted in a near-optimal sensitivity value of 95%. But the SIFT-SVM model performs well and achieved a higher sensitivity value of 96.23%.

The specificity analysis of the SIFT-SVM with compared models is shown in Fig. 12.6. The values in Table 12.2 indicate that the ResNet-50 method has offered the least classifier results by offering the least specificity value of 61%. Then, the VGG-19 model has provided slightly better classifier results by offering a specificity of 68%. Next, the technique devised by Halil et al. leads to a moderate specificity value of 92.68%. Following, the Al-Magni et al. model has resulted in a near-optimal specificity value of 96.69%. Afterward, the Yuan et al. and Li et al. models have resulted to a manageable and near-identical results of 97.50% and 97.80%,

TABLE 12.2

Comparison of Proposed Method with State of the Art Methods

Lasses	Sensitivity	Specificity	Accuracy
SIFT-SVM	**96.23**	**98.16**	**95.42**
VGG-19	95.00	68.00	81.20
ResNet-50	90.00.	61.00	75.50
Yuan et al.	82.50	97.50	93.40
Li et al.	82.00	97.80	93.20
Al-Magni et al.	85.40	96.69	94.03
Halil et al.	90.82	92.68	93.39

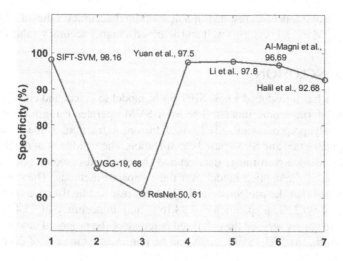

FIGURE 12.6   Comparative results analysis in terms of specificity.

respectively But the SIFT-SVM model performs well and achieved a higher specificity value of 98.16%.

The accuracy analysis of the SIFT-SVM with compared models is shown in Fig. 12.7. The values in Table 12.2 indicate that the ResNet-50 method has offered the least classifier results by offering the least accuracy value of 75.50%. Then, the VGG-19 model has provided slightly better classifier results by offering an accuracy of 81.20%. Next, the technique devised by Li et al. leads to a moderate accuracy value of 93.20%. Afterward, the Halil et al. and Yuan et al. models have resulted in manageable and near-identical results of 93.39% and 93.40%, respectively. Following, the

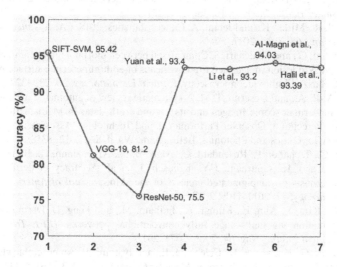

FIGURE 12.7   Comparative results analysis in terms of accuracy.

Al-Magni et al. model has resulted in a near-optimal accuracy value of 94.03%. But the SIFT-SVM model performs well and achieved a higher accuracy value of 95.42%.

12.4 CONCLUSION

This chapter has introduced a new SIFT-SVM model to detect and classify the skin lesion from dermoscopic images. The SIFT-SVM operates using a set of subprocesses namely preprocessing, SIFT-based feature extraction, K-means clustering based segmentation, and SVM-based classification. The validation of the SIFT-SVM takes place using a skin image data set and the obtained outcome pointed out the effectiveness of the applied model over the compared methods. The obtained outcome depicted that the projected SIFT-SVM has resulted in effective results with a sensitivity of 96.23%, a specificity of 98.16%, and an accuracy of 95.42%, respectively. These values verified the enhanced outcome of the proposed model. As a part of future work, the SIFT-SVM model can be improved by the use of deep learning techniques.

REFERENCES

[1] Elmisery, A. M., Rho, S., and Botvich, D., A fog based middleware for automated compliance with OECD privacy principles in internet of healthcare things, *IEEE Access*, 4, 8418–8441, 2016.

[2] Zhang, C., Lai, C. F., Lai, Y. H., Wu, Z. W. and Chao, H. C. An inferential real-time falling posture reconstruction for Internet of healthcare things, *Journal of Network and Computer Applications*, 89, 86–95, 2017.

[3] Feng, J., Isern, N. G., Burton, S. D., and Hu, J. Z. Studies of secondary melanoma on C57BL/6J mouse liver using 1H NMR metabolomics, *Metabolites*, 3, 1011–1035, 2013.

[4] Jemal, A., Siegel, R., Ward, E., Hao, Y., Xu, J., and Thun, M. J. Cancer statistics, 2019, *CA: A Cancer Journal for Clinicians*, 69, 7–34, 2019.

[5] Tarver, T. American Cancer Society. Cancer facts and figures 2014, *Journal of Consumer Health Internet*, 16, 366–367, 2012.

[6] Siegel, R., Miller, K., and Jemal, A. Cancer statistics, 2018. *CA: A Cancer Journal for Clinicians*, 68, 7–30, 2017.

[7] Pellacani, G., and Seidenari, S. Comparison between morphological parameters in pigmented skin lesion images acquired by means of epiluminescence surface microscopy and polarized-light videomicroscopy, *Clinical Dermatology*, 20, 222–227, 2002.

[8] Ali, A.-R. A., and Deserno, T. M. A systematic review of automated melanoma detection in dermatoscopic images and its ground truth data, in Medical Imaging 2012: Image Perception, Observer Performance, and Technology Assessment; International Society for Optics and Photonics: Bellingham, WA, USA, 2012, 8318.

[9] Sinz, C., Tschandl, P., Rosendahl, C., Akay, B. N., Argenziano, G., Blum, A., Braun, R. P., Cabo, H., Gourhant, J.-Y., Kreusch, J., et al. Accuracy of dermatoscopy for the diagnosis of nonpigmented cancers of the skin, *Journal of American Academic Dermatology*, 77, 1100–1109, 2017.

[10] Bi, L., Kim, J., Ahn, E., Kumar, A., Fulham, M., and Feng, D. Dermoscopic image segmentation via multi-stage fully convolutional networks, *IEEE Transactions of Biomedical Engineering*, 64, 2065–2074, 2017.

[11] Schaefer, G., Krawczyk, B., Celebi, M. E., and Iyatomi, H. An ensemble classification approach for melanoma diagnosis, *Memetic Computing*, 6, 233–240, 2014.

[12] Xie, F., and Bovik, A. C. Automatic segmentation of dermoscopy images using self-generating neural networks seeded by genetic algorithm, *Pattern Recognition*, 46, 1012–1019, 2013.

[13] Shankar, K., Lakshmanaprabu, S. K., Gupta, D., Maseleno, A., and De Albuquerque, V. H. C. Optimal feature-based multi-kernel SVM approach for thyroid disease classification, *Journal of Supercomputing*, 1–16, 2018.

[14] Lakshmanaprabu, S. K., Mohanty, S. N., Shankar, K., Arunkumar, N., and Ramirez, G. Optimal deep learning model for classification of lung cancer on CT images, *Future Generation Computer Systems*, 92, 374–382, 2019.

[15] Shankar, K., Elhoseny, M., Lakshmanaprabu, S. K., Ilayaraja, M., Vidhyavathi, R. M., Elsoud, M. A., and Alkhambashi, M. Optimal feature level fusion based ANFIS classifier for brain MRI image classification. *Concurrency and Computation: Practice and Experience*, 32 (1), 1–12, 2018.

[16] Elhoseny, M., and Shankar, K. Optimal bilateral filter and convolutional neural network based denoising method of medical image measurements, *Measurement*, 143, 125–135, 2019.

13 An IoHT-Based Image Compression Model Using Modified Cuckoo Search Algorithm with Vector Quantization

13.1 INTRODUCTION

The rise in development of high-resolution medical images from the Internet of Things (IoT) resulted in the generation of large-sized images. In general, image compression is more important in the multimedia sector. Recently, the introduction of image compression methods with optimized reformed image quality has been one of the significant operations for several developers [1, 2]. The main aim of image compression is for transmitting images with lower bits. Exploring redundancies from an image, applicable encoding models, as well as conversion methods are assumed to be the major aspects present in image compression. The initial image compression approach was presented by a team named the Joint Photographic Experts Group (JPEG). Quantization is of two types: scalar quantization and vector quantization (VQ). It is referred to as a nontransformed compression, which is an effective tool applied in lossy image compression. The intention of VQ is to develop a productive codebook with a collection of codewords where the input image is declared based on the lower Euclidean distance.

Initially, the constantly employed VQ model is the Linde–Buzo–Gray (LBG) approach (1980). It is defined as easy, applicable, and stable, and also depends upon the lower Euclidean distance among image vectors and adjacent codewords. It generates a local optimal solution, but it cannot ensure excellent global solutions. The LBG model's solution is based on the primary codebook produced randomly. Patane and Russo presented an enhanced LBG (ELBG) technique that boosts the local optimized solution of the LBG method [3]. The fundamental suggestion of ELBG is an effective application of codewords; a productive tool applied for resolving major limitations involved in clustering methods and reaches a good result when compared with LBG, which is autonomous at the initial codebook.

Projection VQ (PVQ) employs the quadtree (QT) decomposition to divide the image as variable-sized blocks that denote by single orientation reconstruction (SOR) and it demonstrates the enhanced function of subjective and objective abilities related with permanent-sized blocks. Object-relied VQ is classified into three stages: initialization, iterative, and finalization. First, the initialization stage depends upon the Max–Min technique. Alternatively, the iteration stage is referred to as an adaptive LBG approach. Finally, finalization eliminates the redundancy from a codebook. A QT decomposing technique enables VQ with different block size by monitoring homogeneity of the local area; however, Kazuya et al. (2008) tracked that complexity of local areas of an image is required when compared with homogeneity [4]. Thus, a VQ of images along with variable block size that quantifies complex regions of the image under the application of Local Fractal Dimensions (LFDs) has been projected.

Dimitrios et al. [5] deployed a fuzzy VQ in image compression that relied on a competing agglomeration and new codeword migration procedure; a learning approach for developing fuzzy clustering–based VQ under the combination of three learning phases. Therefore, a multivariate VQ (MVQ) technology has been employed to compress hyperspectral imagery (HSI). The efficient codebook is deployed with the help of fuzzy c-mean (FCM). Hence, the attained results show that MVQ performs quite well when compared with traditional VQ by mean squared error (MSE) and reformed image quality. Wang and Meng [6] monitored that image compression could be operated with converted VQ where the image that has to be quantized is converted with a discrete wavelet transform (DWT).

Recently, soft computation models have been deployed in the applications of engineering and scientific issues. Rajpoot et al. [7] developed a codebook under the employment of the Ant Colony Optimization (ACO) scheme. The codebook was designed by applying ACO by showing wavelet coefficient from a bidirectional graph and describing the applicable approach to place the edges on a graph with maximum convergence. Hence, Tsaia et al. [8] projected a rapid ACO in codebook generation under the observation of repeated evaluations of the ACO method. The speed of convergence in ACO can be improved by finding redundant estimations while developing a codebook and it is evident than ACO has failed to achieve better convergence. Additionally, particle swarm optimization (PSO) VQ depends upon the improvement of particle global best (gbest) and local best (pbest) solutions and performs a better LBG technique. The gbest is comprised of higher fitness rates between populations and pbest has optimal fitness measure of adjacent values.

Feng et al. [9] implied that evolutionary fuzzy PSO models are composed with an optimal global codebook and the working function is better when compared with PSO and LBG techniques. Quantum particle swarm optimization (QPSO) is presented by Wang [10] to resolve the 0–1 knapsack problem and enhance the function of PSO. The QPSO process is more optimal than PSO; it evaluates the local points from pbest and gbest for every particle and upgrades the location of the particle by selecting proper variables u that are from the arbitrary value from the range of (0,1) and z denotes the nonnegative constant which lies in the range of 0 to 2.8. Chang et al. [11] applied a tree-shaped VQ to deploy a codebook model using triangle inequality to attain effective codewords along with higher convergence duration. Therefore, Yu-Chen et al. [12] implied a rapid codebook search method that applies two test conditions to improve the image encoding strategy with no additional image distortion. Based on the simulation results, the maximum reduction in the implementation time could be reached if there is a codebook of 256 codewords.

Sanyal et al. [13] presented a novel method in choosing chemotaxis phases of the fundamental Bacterial Foraging Optimization Algorithm (BFOA) that tends to design a closer optimized codebook in image compression with best reformed image quality as well as higher peak signal-to-noise ratio. It selects a fuzzy membership function (MF) as an objective function that has been optimized under the application of extended BFOA when compared with the results of alternate optimizing methods. Horng and Jiang [14] used honeybee mating optimization approach (HBMO) for VQ. HBMO is comprised of high qualified reformed images and a better codebook with minimum distortion when compared with PSO-LBG, QPSO-LBG, and LBG approaches. Horng [15] utilized a Firefly (FF) technique to develop a codebook in VQ.

The FF model is inspired by the social events of fireflies with the presence of bioluminescent interaction. FFs have minimum brighter intensity rates that move in the direction of brighter intensity fireflies. The FA faces a problem if there is an absence of brighter fireflies in the search space, thus Chiranjeevi et al. [16] projected an extended FA where fireflies employ particular procedures if there is a lack of brighter fireflies in the search space. Chiranjeevi and Jena [17] employed a bat optimization algorithm (BA) to develop an effective codebook with proper selection of tuning parameters as well as evident PSNR performance as well as the convergence duration when compared with FA. Also, a color image undergoes compression using VQ under actual data in prior demosaicking and process mosaicking to reform the RGB bands.

A new VQ method to encode the wavelet decomposed color image under the application of the Modified Artificial Bee Colony (ABC) approach and the accomplished results were compared with genetic algorithm (GA) and normal ABC with the benchmark LBG model and the simulation outcome shows a maximum PSNR reconstruction [18]. The presented technique is employed with the cuckoo search (CS) for developing an effective codebook that generates optimal VQ and tends to a higher peak signal-to-noise ratio (PSNR) with better reformed image quality. The CS method is more suitable for increasing or decreasing the linear and nonlinear issues. Here, an MCS technology is applied for effective codebook development. The parameter setting of PSO, QPSO, HBMO, and FA is assumed to be a critical operation with ineffective tuning parameters influencing the function of models. The CS approach is elegant and comprised of two tuning parameters: skewness and mutation probability. The method performs well when compared with PSO, QPSO, HBMO, and FA for linear and nonlinear mathematical optimizing issues.

The effectiveness of the compression technique is solely based on the quantization table and the selection of the quantization table is considered as an optimization issue that can be resolved using bio-inspired algorithms. This chapter presents a new MCS-based LBG algorithm to compress the images generated by IoT devices. The MCS is an extension of classical CSA by modifying the intensification and diversification models. A brief set of simulation takes place and the results are examined under diverse aspects. The proposed MCS-LBG model has resulted in optimal compression performance over compared methods.

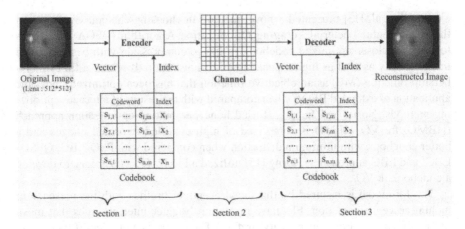

FIGURE 13.1 Encoding and decoding process of VQ.

13.2 VECTOR QUANTIZATION AND LBG ALGORITHM

Here, VQ has been experimented at three phases: encoder, channel, and decoder. The architecture of VQ is depicted in Fig. 13.1. The structure is constrained with three blocks where every block is comprised of diverse operating strategies. Block 1 is named as the encoder section. Image vectors can be produced by dividing an input image into adverse as well as nonoverlapping blocks. The origination of an effective codebook is the major operation in VQ. A codebook is composed of a collection of codewords of a size similar to a nonoverlapping block size. This model is named as an optimized one when the produced codebook is effective. Once a productive codebook is generated, every vector undergoes indexing with the help of the index value acquired from the index table. Block 2 is a channel by which indexed values can be forwarded to a receiver. Block 3 is a decoder section that encloses an index table, codebook, and reformed image. Hence, received indexed values undergo decoding with the receiver index table. The codebook that exists at the receiver is similar to the transmitter codebook.

The frequently used VQ in the LBG-VQ model is Generalized Lloyd Algorithm (GLA) termed as LBG approach. The distortion is reduced after implementing the LBG technique and offers a local codebook. The following steps are given below and also shown in Fig. 13.2:

1. Load with initial codebook C_1 of size N. Assume the iteration value as $m = 1$ and initial distortion $D_1 = \infty$.
2. By applying codebook $C_m = \{Y_i\}$, partition the training set as cluster sets R_i with the application of the nearest neighbor condition.
3. After the mapping of input vectors to initial code vectors is computed, determine the centroids of the partition area found in Step 2. It provides an enhanced codebook C_{m+1}.
4. Estimate the average distortion D_{m+1}. If $D_m - D_{m+1} < T$ then terminates, else $m = m + 1$ and follow Step 2 to Step 4.

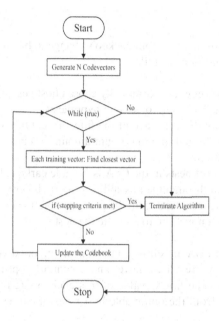

FIGURE 13.2   Overall process of the LBG algorithm.

13.3   PROPOSED MCS-LBG ALGORITHM–BASED VQ

Fig. 13.3 shows the processes involved in the MCS-LBG algorithm for VQ. Initially, the original image is partitioned into nonoverlapping blocks. Then, the codebook generation takes place by the MCS-LBG algorithm. Then, the encoded data will be transmitted by the use of the indexing table. Then, the encoded data will be transmitted and is decoded by the use of the indexing table. Finally, the decoded data will be reconstructed by the use of the MCS-LBG algorithm.

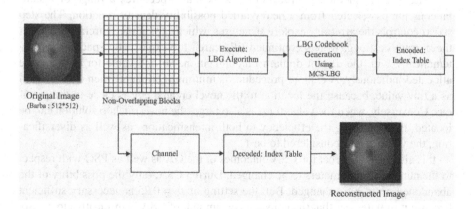

FIGURE 13.3   Overall process of the MCS-LBG model.

13.3.1 CS Algorithm

The CSA that draws simulation from cuckoo's change to breeding and replication is perfected by the suppositions as follows:

- All cuckoos lay 1 egg in an arbitrarily chosen host nest at a time, as the egg signifies the feasible result to issue in hypothesis;
- The CSA follows the existence of the fittest rule. Only the fittest between every host nest through the maximum amount of eggs are accepted on to the next generation;
- The amount of host nests in the CSA is suitable early. A host bird spots the intruder solution through the possibility $p_a \in [0,1]$. For such conditions, the host bird is either removed from the parasitic solution or abandons the nest entirely to seek a novel site to recreate the nest.

The steps involved in CSA are elitism, intensification, and diversification. Initially, a population of feasible results, a novel and potentially optimal solution (cuckoo egg) is created. When the fitness value of this cuckoo egg is high and arbitrarily choose the solutions from the obtainable host nests, it can be exchanged with the worst egg.

A cuckoo lays an egg at an arbitrary position using Levy flight that is characterized with

$$x_i = (iter + 1) = x_i (iter) + \alpha \times \text{lévy}(\lambda), \tag{13.1}$$

$$levy \ (\lambda) = | \frac{\Gamma(1+\lambda) \times \sin (\pi\lambda/2)}{\Gamma((1+\lambda)/2) \times \lambda \times 2^{((\lambda-1)/2)}} |^{1/\lambda} \tag{13.2}$$

where x_i is the feasible egg, *iter* indicates the present generation number, Γ is the gamma function that is determined with the integral: $\Gamma(x) = \int_0^\infty e^{-t} t^{x-1} \, dt$, and λ is a constant $(1 < \lambda \leq 3)$.

A Levy flight method is an arbitrary walk that procedures a range of instantaneous jumps selected from a heavy-tailed possibility density function. The step size α controls the arbitrary explore structures, which exploit the search space about the current best egg. It gets continued till search the exploration space more systematically with the distant domain randomization. So, the value for α should be allocated judiciously. A explore procedure is minimum efficient when α is selected as a tiny value, because the location to the novel created egg is close to the previous. Conversely, when the value for α is also large, the novel cuckoo solution can be located. For balancing the efficiency to both intensifications as well as diversification, the value of α is considered to be 1.

It is also indicated that the CSA outcomes of the GA as well as PSO with respect to the number of parameters to be changed. During CSA, only the possibility of the abandoned nests p_a is changed. But, the setting of $p_a = 0.25$ is necessary sufficient because it initiates out that the convergence amount of CSA is insensitive to p_a. So, the fraction of nests to desert p_a is considered as 0.25.

13.3.2 MCS ALGORITHM

In an optimized manner, determining the optimal results competently as well as correctly greatly relies on the essential explore method. The efficiency of the usual CSA is unquestionable, meaning that if provided sufficient calculation time, it can eventually be guaranteed to meet for optimum eggs. But the search procedure found to be time consuming because of the connection arbitrary walk behavior. To enhance the rate of convergence as preserving the eye-catching features of the CSA, an accelerated exploring method also is presented by the incorporation of the inertia weight control approach in the PSO.

The step size α that controls the local as well as global exploring is allocated as constant in the usual CSA, where $\alpha = 1$ is performed. During the present work, a novel adaptive cuckoo search algorithm (ACSA) is proposed. In place of utilizing a constant value, the stage size α is changed adaptively in the presented ACSA, depending on the hypothesis that the cuckoos lay their solutions at the area through a maximum solution rate of survival. Considering, with changing the stage size α adaptively, cuckoos explore the present optimal egg to lay a solution as this area is feasible is contain the best eggs, then, on the contrary, they search more rigorously to an optimal situation when the present habitat is not appropriate for breeding. The phase size α is defined adaptively as follows:

$$\alpha = \begin{cases} \alpha_L + (\alpha_U - \alpha_L)\dfrac{F_j - F_{\min}}{F_{avg} - F_{\min}}, & F_j > F_{avg} \\ \dfrac{\alpha_U}{\sqrt{t}}, & F_j \le F_{avg}, \end{cases} \tag{13.3}$$

where α_L is the already less step size, α_U is the existing high step size, F_j is the fitness value of the *jth* cuckoo solution, and $F_{\min}$ and F_{avg} indicate the less and average fitness values of every host nest, correspondingly.

The step size α defines distance of the novel cuckoo solution from the present host nest. Determining the less and high Levy flight step size values correctly is vital such that the explore method in the ACSA is neither aggressive nor too useless. The α_L and α_M are selected depending on the field of x_1. In addition, as a precautionary quantity, when ACSA create a cuckoo solution that decreases the external field of interest, its location is endured unaltered.

13.3.3 WORKING PROCESS OF MCS-LBG ALGORITHM

A block representation of VQ utilizing a CS technique is depicted in Fig. 13.3. The VQ is separated into direct and nonoverlapping blocks. A created codebook of LBG technique is optimized by the CS technique which assures the globe convergence rate. Besides, CS is capable to explore the local codebook as well as global codebook to control the mutation probability (P_a).

A CS technique works through subsequent three idealized principles: All cuckoos lays 1 solution at a time, and dump it in an arbitrarily selected nest; an optimal nest through a maximum amount of eggs is taken up by the next generations; the amount of available host nests is suitable, and a host has defined an alien solution through a possibility $P_a \in [0, 1]$. On the other hand, a host bird is either thrown the solution

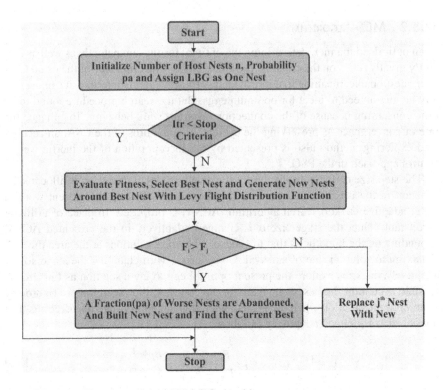

FIGURE 13.4 Flowchart of the MCS-LBG algorithm.

missing or abandons the nest to create an entirely novel nest in a novel position. Now every cuckoo nest is considered as a codebook. The flowchart of the MCS technique is reviewed in Fig. 13.4. A described technique to vector quantizes is as follows:

i. (Primary of parameters and eggs): Set the count of host nests through all nests to have a single solution, mutation probability (P_a), and acceptance. Run the LBG technique as well as allocate its result as one of the nest/ solutions and rest nests arbitrarily.

ii. (Chosen the present optimal egg): To compute the fitness of every nest as well as choose the highest fitness nest as the present best nest $nest_{best}$.

iii. (Create novel eggs by Mantegna's method): Novel cuckoo nests $(nest_{new})$ are created that are present best nests by arbitrary walk (Levy flight). During the arbitrary walk, subsequent Levy distribution function accepts Mantegna's technique. A novel nest is provided as

$$nest_{new} = nest_{old} + \alpha \otimes l\acute{e}vy(\lambda) \qquad (13.4)$$

where a is the phase size generally corresponding to one as well as Levy; (k) is the Levy distribution function

iv. (Discard worst nets and exchange by novel nests): When the created arbitrary number (K) is larger than the mutation probability (P_a) next exchange poor nests through novel nests with retaining the optimal nest unmodified. A novel nest is created with an arbitrary walk as well as an arbitrary phase size is provided as

$$nest_{new} = nest_{old} + (K \times setpsize) \tag{13.5}$$

where

$$setpsize = r \times (nest_{rand} - nest_{rand})(r \ is \ random \ number) \tag{13.6}$$

v. Position the nests depending on fitness function and choose the better nest.
vi. Replicate Step 2 to Step 4 until the end condition.

13.4 PERFORMANCE VALIDATION

For investigating the results of the presented MCS-LBG algorithm, a detailed validation of the results takes place on the benchmark medical images as illustrated in Fig. 13.5 [9]. The different kinds of medicinal images employed for evaluation are diabetic retinopathy, diatom, and mammographic images. To ensure the effectual performance of the proposed model, extensive analysis has been carried out. For ensuring effective results on the compression performance, the visual quality of the reconstructed images takes place.

Table 13.1 and Fig. 13.6 show the results offered by the MCS-LBG algorithm on the applied test images in terms of space savings (SS). The table values indicated that the MCS-LBG algorithm achieves maximal SS over the compared methods. On the applied 13_left image, it is observed that the MCS-LBG algorithm achieves a maximum SS of 95.43% whereas the existing CS and discrete cosine transform (DCT) models lead to slightly lower SS of 92.30% and 86.49%, respectively. Similarly,

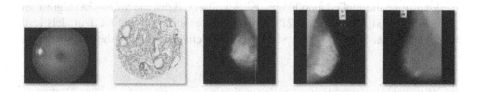

FIGURE 13.5 Sample test images.

TABLE 13.1
Comparative SS Analysis of Distinct Models

Images Name	MCS-LBG	CS	DCT
13_left	95.43	92.30	86.49
A_4_12_4096	94.30	91.48	85.20
mdb001	94.82	92.49	84.20
mdb004	95.20	93.98	89.02
mdb005	94.21	93.09	91.37
Average	**94.79**	**92.67**	**87.26**

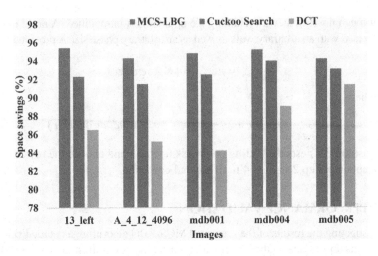

FIGURE 13.6   SS analysis of diverse models.

on the applied A_4_12_4096 image, it is observed that the MCS-LBG algorithm achieves a maximum SS of 94.30% whereas the existing CS and DCT models lead to slightly lower SS of 91.48% and 85.20%, respectively. Likewise, on the applied mdb001 image, it is observed that the MCS-LBG algorithm achieves a maximum SS of 94.82% whereas the existing CS and DCT models lead to slightly lower SS of 92.49% and 84.20%, respectively. Along with that, on the applied mdb004 image, it is observed that the MCS-LBG algorithm achieves a maximum SS of 95.20% whereas the existing CS and DCT models lead to slightly lower SS of 93.98% and 89.02%, respectively.

Finally, on the applied mdb005 image, it is observed that the MCS-LBG algorithm achieves a maximum SS of 94.21% whereas the existing CS and DCT models lead to slightly lower SS of 93.09% and 91.37%, respectively. Fig. 13.7 shows the average

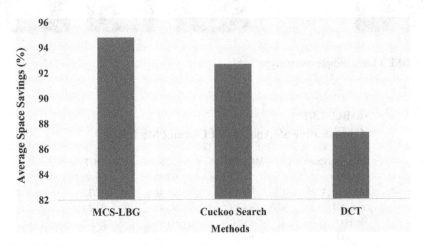

FIGURE 13.7   Average SS analysis of diverse models.

TABLE 13.2

Comparison of Proposed Methods with Existing Methods in Terms of PSNR

Images Name	MCS-LBG	Cuckoo Search	DCT
13_left	54.39	43.22	40.29
A_4_12_4096	50.23	45.30	39.40
mdb001	49.29	47.20	42.49
mdb004	47.39	43.87	40.86
mdb005	50.47	42.40	38.22
Average	**50.35**	**44.39**	**40.25**

SS analysis of distinct models. On average, it is mentioned that the MCS-LBG algorithm has shown its effective compression performance by attaining a maximum SS of 94.79% whereas a lower average SS of 92.67% and 87.26% has been achieved by the existing CS and DCT models.

Table 13.2 and Fig. 13.8 shows the results offered by the MCS-LBG algorithm on the applied test images in terms of SS. The table values indicated that the MCS-LBG algorithm achieves maximal PSNR over the compared methods. On the applied 13_left image, it is observed that the MCS-LBG algorithm achieves a maximum PSNR of 54.39 dB whereas the existing CS and DCT models lead to a slightly lower PSNR of 43.22 dB and 40.29 dB, respectively. Similarly, on the applied A_4_12_4096 image, it is observed that the MCS-LBG algorithm achieves a maximum PSNR of 50.23 dB whereas the existing CS and DCT models lead to a slightly lower PSNR of 45.30 dB and 39.40 dB, respectively. Likewise, on the applied mdb001 image, it is observed that the MCS-LBG algorithm achieves a maximum PSNR of 49.29 dB whereas the existing CS and DCT models lead to a slightly lower PSNR of 47.20 dB and 42.49 dB, respectively. Along with that, on the applied mdb004 image, it is observed that the MCS-LBG algorithm achieves a maximum PSNR of 47.39 dB

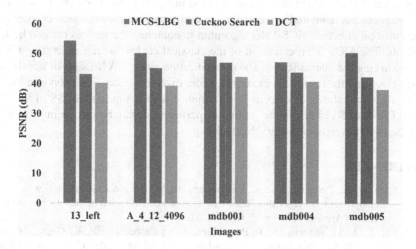

FIGURE 13.8 PSNR analysis of diverse models.

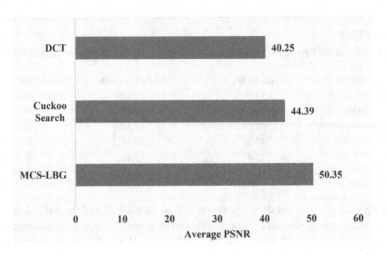

FIGURE 13.9   Average PSNR analysis of diverse models.

whereas the existing CS and DCT models lead to a slightly lower PSNR of 43.87 dB and 40.86 dB, respectively.

Finally, on the applied mdb005 image, it is observed that the MCS-LBG algorithm achieves a maximum PSNR of 50.47 dB whereas the existing CS and DCT models lead to a slightly lower PSNR of 42.40 dB and 38.22 dB, respectively. Fig. 13.9 shows the average PSNR analysis of distinct models. On average, it is mentioned that the MCS-LBG algorithm has shown its effective compression performance by attaining a maximum PSNR of 50.35 dB whereas a lower average PSNR of 44.39 dB and 40.25 dB has been achieved by the existing CS and DCT models.

13.5   CONCLUSION

In general, the efficiency of any compression model depends upon the selection of the quantization table and is treated as an optimization problem. This chapter has presented an effective MCS-LBG algorithm to compress the images created by IoT gadgets. The MCS is an extension of the classical cuckoo search algorithm (CSA) by modifying the intensification and diversification models. A brief set of simulation takes place and the results are examined under diverse aspects. The proposed MCS-LBG algorithm shows its effective performance with the maximum SS of 94.79% and a PSNR of 50.35 dB. In the future, the performance can be further improved by the use of lightweight cryptographic techniques.

REFERENCES

[1] Shankar, K., Perumal, E., and Vidhyavathi, R. M. Deep neural network with moth search optimization algorithm based detection and classification of diabetic retinopathy images, *SN Applied Sciences*, 2(4), 1–10, 2020.

[2] Raj, R. J. S., Shobana, S. J., Pustokhina, I. V., Pustokhin, D. A., Gupta, D., and Shankar, K. Optimal feature selection-based medical image classification using deep learning model in Internet of Medical Things, *IEEE Access*, 8, 58006–58017, 2020.

[3] Patane, G., and Russo, M. The enhanced LBG algorithm, *Neural Networks*, 14, 1219–1237, 2002.

[4] Kazuya, S., Sato, S., Junji, M., and Yukinori, S. Vector quantization of images with variable block size, *Applied Soft Computing*, 8, 634–645, 2008.

[5] Dimitrios, T., George, E. T., and John, T. Fuzzy vector quantization for image compression based on competitive agglomeration and a novel codeword migration strategy, *Engineering Applied Artificial Intelligence*, 25, 1212–1225, 2012.

[6] Wang, X., and Meng, J. A 2-D ECG compression algorithm based on wavelet transform and vector quantization, *Digital Signal Process,* 18, 179–188, 2008.

[7] Rajpoot, A., Hussain, A., Saleem, K., and Qureshi, Q. A novel image coding algorithm using ant colony system vector quantization, in International workshop on systems, signals and image processing, Poznan, Poland, 2004.

[8] Tsaia, C. W., Tsengb, S. P., Yang, C. S., and Chiang, M. C. PREACO: a fast ant colony optimization for codebook generation, *Applied Soft Computing,* 13, 3008–3020, 2013.

[9] Feng, H., Chen, C., and Fun, Y. Evolutionary fuzzy particle swarm optimization vector quantization learning scheme in image compression. *Expert Systems with Applications,* 32, 213–222, 2007.

[10] Wang, Y., Feng, X. Y., Huang, Y. X., Zhou, W. G., and Liang, Y. C. A novel quantum swarm evolutionary algorithm and its applications, *Neurocomputing,* 70, 633–640, 2007.

[11] Chang, C., Li, Y. C., and Yeh, J. Fast codebook search algorithms based on tree-structured vector quantization, *Pattern Recognition Letters*, 27, 1077–86, 2006.

[12] Yu-Chen, H., Bing, H., and Chih, C. T. Fast VQ codebook search for gray scale image coding, *Image and Vision Computing*, 26, 657–666, 2008.

[13] Sanyal, N., Chatterjee, A., and Munshi, S. Modified bacterial foraging optimization technique for vector quantization-based image compression, in Computational Intelligence in Image Processing, Springer, 2013, 131–152.

[14] Horng, M., and Jiang, T. Image vector quantization algorithm via honey bee mating optimization, *Expert Systems with Applications*, 38, 1382–1392, 2011.

[15] Horng, M. Vector quantization using the firefly algorithm for image compression, *Expert Systems with Applications,* 39, 1078–1091, 2012.

[16] Chiranjeevi, K., Jena, U. R., Murali, B., and Jeevan, K. Modified firefly algorithm (MFA) based vector quantization for image compression, *Computational Intelligence in Data Mining (ICCIDM), Advance in Intelligent Systems and Computing*, 2, 373–381, 2015.

[17] Chiranjeevi, K., and Jena, U. R. Fast vector quantization using bat algorithm for image compression, *International Journal of Engineering Science Technology*, 19, 769–781, 2016.

[18] Lakshmia, M., Senthilkumar, J., and Suresh, Y. Visually lossless compression for Bayer color filter array using optimized Vector Quantization, *Applied Soft Computing,* 46, 1030–1042, 2016.

14 An Effective Secure Medical Image Transmission Using Improved Particle Swarm Optimization and Wavelet Transform

14.1 INTRODUCTION

Internet of Things (IoT) devices are commonly employed for interconnecting existing medicinal sources and offer a reliable, efficient, and intelligent healthcare service to ageing patients with chronic illnesses. Magnetic resonance imaging (MRI) is filled with various advantages when compared with alternate medical imaging models and plays a vital role in neuroscience study and common neurotic anomaly detection. It contains differential points of interest to apply the imaging in diverse methods since it is capable of showing the action of the human brain [1]. Moreover, it is more secure if it is contrasted with alternate imaging methods. Hence, several approaches are presented to analyze MRI data [2]. The symptomatic evaluations of MRI are developed under the application of programmed as well as the accurate separation of MRI images.

Recently, many developers have projected various methodologies to attain the desired goal. In previous decades, various methodologies have been applied to realize the neurotic brain. In the case of dividing MRI images, the application of patient information should meet the congruity among data usage and computing capable failure due to the unintentional distribution of personal details. This is referred to as a promising application to develop a novel approach for secured Internet of Medical Things (IoMT) [3], which ensures the legal accessing and application of patient's data. The privacy of a patient's private data has become endangered by digital health details that are distributed across insecure teams. It provides a negative impact on patients as well as legitimate parties. Therefore, the security of patient's data is a challenging factor for developers to apply these data in a finite analyzing process.

The recently identified quantum process of IoMT in healthcare segments is related to the healthcare of a patient, which is comprised of mobility and makes

163

a vulnerable network for diverse kinds of attacks. Therefore, the security, privacy, trustworthiness, and simultaneously of a patient's therapeutic as well as sensitive details are named as a potential challenge in the healthcare platform. In [4], a new method to tackle patient's secured information, a discrete wavelet transform (DWT) technique, has been presented to apply permanence as well as self-sufficiency characteristics of the blockchain. Furthermore, modification of clashing interests to ensure privacy at the time of providing permission to apply data in legit purposes for analyzing process is discussed. To assure the privacy of patients Electronic Health Records (EHRs) and motivate the aforementioned trade-off, only a few methods are mentioned in [5].

Privacy-conserving technologies focus on counteracting divulgence of simple personal data, at the time of developing affected data applied in licit problems. There are diverse experiments carried out for sensitive data integrity that should be transformed to provide a ground-breaking impact on the concerned problem. The application of such models enables the interchange among data security and classification, to provide data usage to limit the malicious breach in data security. The combination of IoT and data transmission makes a vital tool with effective analyzing ability to ensure the security of patient's data. Since the medical images are enclosed with patients' personalized information, privacy protection has increased amid transmitting clinical images through the web [6]. Therefore, steganography is applied for providing privacy as well as confidentiality by protecting the private information of patients from therapeutic images.

The study ensures privacy and security of patient's therapeutic data and finds the data that has not been acquired. On the other hand, it attains a desired classification value, with extra details in the computer-aided diagnosis (CAD) technique. For accomplishing this process, the deployed model uses steganography to cover the personal data of a patient inside an MRI system before undergoing medical analysis. Therefore, it is applied with spatial domain image steganography to incorporate patients' information and research on a state-of-the-art mechanism where it applies a generic and common steganography system.

The modified image along with a slight color difference is expected to be indistinguishable. Researchers have tried to explore the applicable positions to develop an embed highest invisible method. Yang et al. [7] have employed a least significant bits (LSB) substitution-relied hiding that resolves noise-sensitive areas to attain optimal visual quality as well as the smoothing fact of the stego image (SI). In [8], protective data transmission of sensitive contents across the Internet as attained by dual-level security, which can be reached by cyclic18 LSB substitution on encrypted images, is discussed. Finally, the simulation outcome of this method offers good imperceptibility and security.

In [9], the projected multi-pixel differencing (MPD) and LSB steganographic procedure to incorporate the private data with edges and smooth blocks is discussed. Muhammad et al. [10] implied a secured image steganographic procedure where secret data undergoes encryption with the application of a multi-level encryption model, and embeds from a cover image by applying the stego key directed adaptive LSB substitution. Consequently, in [11], researchers proposed an approach in LSB substitution to combine more volume of payload on edges of the image.

Muhammad et al. [12] have deployed the Magic LSB Substitution Method (M-LSB-SM)-relied steganographic framework to corporate the secret data on the cover image. The cover image is transformed from red green blue (RGB) to hue saturation intensity (HSI) colorspace to attain encrypted secret details.

Laskar and Hemachandran [13] employed a transposition cipher-based cryptography on payload before forwarding to an LSB substitution steganography on the cover image. Joo et al. [14] projected a pixel-value differencing (PVD) mechanism that applies floor and modulus function to provide optimal security from attackers. Rahim et al. [15] deployed a private data protection module under the application of deep autoencoder (DAE) for rapid image retrieving mobile devices. The developed model ensures easy image retrieval on the application of the latest mobile devices. Only some of the analyzes to use image steganography on security and legitimacy of visual social media are demonstrated. In [16], a discrete cosine transform (DCT) relying on a data covering principle has been deployed for concealing color data from gray-level images. It is evident that the image steganographic method applying the LSB substitution procedure is utilized in many types of research due to enough alarming efficiency. An easy embed method could be used with various data types. The image pixels presented in a spatial domain can be modified to attain secret data. Higher imperceptibility and capacity are fundamental in ensuring secured transmission of secret data. The LSB of the cover image has been embedded with bits of secret message.

This study introduces an improved particle swarm optimization (IPSO)-DWT approach to effectively select the pixels to embed the secret image. The IPSO-DWT algorithm makes use of fitness function (FF), with respect to cost function (CF). The CF evaluates the fitness based on the determination of the edge, entropy, and pixel intensities to validate FF. An elaborate experimental analysis takes place to validate the goodness of the IPSO-DWT algorithm. The results ensured the optimal outcome of the IPSO-DWT algorithm in terms of mean square error (MSE) and peak signal to noise ratio (PSNR) over compared methods.

14.2 THE IPSO-DWT METHOD

This chapter presents the cost-relied IPSO method that depends upon the extension of the IPSO method. Hence, the projected approach steganographic investigation of the image by the developed IPSO technique. The image steganography offers optimal security and the ability of securing protective messages from being attacked. The presented approach applies a sparse approach to enhance the image security. Fig. 14.1 depicts the block diagram of the presented model. It can attain the image steganography in two phases: embed and extraction. The incorporating of the image acquires the cover image as well as the secret image. The cover image is defined as the process that is treated as a stego key. After the completion of the secret message, IDWT can be employed to show the image in the spatial domain. In the next stage, the secret image extraction process takes place where the embed image is converted into spatial as well as frequency domains. Followed by, the sparse signal has been filtered and is applied to obtain a secret image.

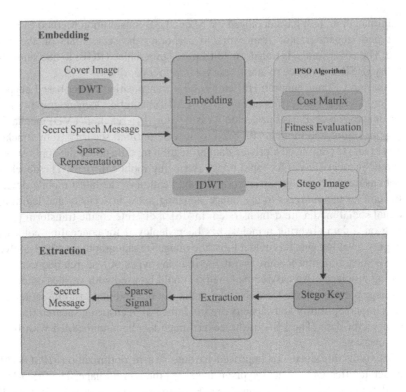

FIGURE 14.1 Block diagram of the IPSO-DWT method.

14.2.1 EMBEDDED PROCEDURE

There are diverse phases in the embed model: at the initial stage, the stego key, as well as the secret image, are attained and the length of the secret image. Following, the process of DWT to filter the wavelet of higher and lower frequencies. Next, pick up the wavelet coefficient from obtained wavelet; along with choosing the pixels for making fit in embed. An optimized location for the embedded procedure is computed with the application of PSO to select patterns that select an appropriate perfect pixel to incorporate the secret message. Next, the secret message is embedded with extended coefficients and combined unmodified coefficients. Consequently, the formation of the SI where it applies IDWT. The task of the embedded procedure is depicted in Fig. 14.2.

14.2.1.1 Representation of the Stego Key

This module applies the cover image as a stego key. Also, it is defined as applied to hide the sensitive data. The stego key is the actual image where the message signal undergoes embed. The embed task repeats in the cover image with no alteration in the statistical parameters of the cover image. Assume the cover image as C with the dimension $P \times Q$. The band coefficients of getting subsampling and DWT is provided by

$$[C_1 C_2 C_3 C_4] = DWT(C) \tag{14.1}$$

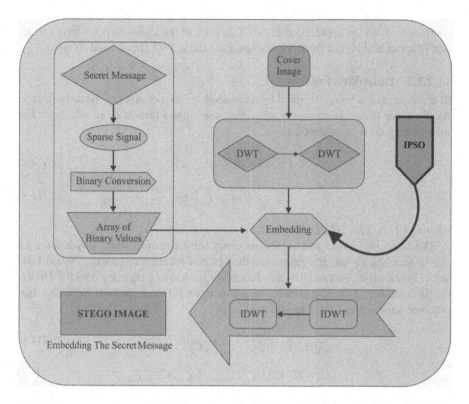

FIGURE 14.2 Embedded procedure.

where C_1 implies the coefficient of minimum frequency, which holds vital data of an image, i.e., proper bands; C_2, C_3, and C_4 are referred as coefficients of an insignificant wavelet that captures data and mimics the texture as well as the edge of the image, i.e., higher frequency bands. Every obtained sample is dimension $j \times k$, correspondingly. The bands chosen for the further process are C_1 and C_4, i.e., coefficients of minimum and maximum frequency bands. Under the application of DWT to C_1 and C_4, sub-bands obtained from C_1 and C_4 are given as

$$[C_1^{LL} C_1^{LH} C_1^{HL} C_1^{HH}] = DWT(C_1) \tag{14.2}$$

$$[C_4^{LL} C_4^{LH} C_4^{HL} C_4^{HH}] = DWT(C_4) \tag{14.3}$$

where C_1^{LL} and C_4^{LL} are minimum frequency sub-bands of coefficients C_1 and C_4 correspondingly, $C_1^{LH}, C_1^{HL}, C_1^{HH}$ are named as maximum frequency sub-bands of C_1, and $C_4^{LH}, C_4^{HL}, C_4^{HH}$ are greater frequency sub-bands produced from C_4. It is evident that the minimum frequency band gives each vital data of the image and maximum frequency bands produce the texture and edge data of the image. The dimensions of every sub-band are produced from bands C_1 and C_4 is $\left(\dfrac{j}{2} \times \dfrac{l_t}{2} \right)$. The obtained band coefficients with the application of DWT are due to the enabling pixel-wise extraction of lower and higher frequency bands and offers DWT the desired solution.

14.2.1.2 Embedded Process

SI is a consequent image attained by embedded secret messages to the cover image. As the cover image is named as stego key, the embed task is more effective. The modified signal is represented as

$$C_1^{*j} = C_1^j + (S_i \cdot P_{opt} \cdot \alpha) \tag{14.4}$$

$$C_4^j = C_4^j + (S_i \cdot P_{opt} \cdot \alpha) \tag{14.5}$$

where $j = \{LL, LH, HL, HH\}; 1 \le i \le 8$

The norm j is a lower and higher frequency sub-band of C_1 and C_4, S_j denotes the sparse message signal, P_{opt} represents the optimal location to process embed task, and α implies the constant. The sub-bands are named as frequency domain. Hence, the presentation of the image in the spatial domain is the essential IDWT. The final outcome attained by IDWT can be defined by

$$C_1^* = IDWT(C_1^{*LL}, C_1^{*LH}, C_1^{*HL}, C_1^{*HH}) \tag{14.6}$$

$$C_4^* = IDWT(C_4^{*LL}, C_4^{*LH}, C_4^{*HL}, C_4^{*HH}) \tag{14.7}$$

Hence, the embed signal with extended bands C_1 and C_4 is

$$C^* = IDWT(C_1^*, C_2, C_3, C_4^*) \tag{14.8}$$

14.2.2 EXTRACTION OF THE SECRET MESSAGE

The process of extracting an efficient hidden message from SI is named as a secret image. The SI is provided as input to the embed process, which is carried out on the reception side. The SI has been processed using DWT for converting spatial presentation of SI into the frequency domain. Later, the sparse signal is obtained from SI, which is transformed in binary format, and the secret images are filtered. The input for the extraction process is in the format of SI, referred to as C^{*E}. This SI is present in a spatial domain. However, DWT can apply to representing SI in the frequency domain with higher and lower frequency bands. These coefficients compute different variables such as edge, texture, and significant information of image. Therefore, coefficients of bands are produced in the form of a result for DWT as

$$\left[C_1^{*E} C_2^{*E} C_3^{*E} C_4^{*E} \right] = DWT(C^{*E}) \tag{14.9}$$

where $C_1^{*E}, C_2^{*E}, C_3^{*E}$, and C_4^{*E} are the coefficients of the bands produced under the application of DWT and C^{*E} is a SI, that is referred as a secret message embedded in a cover image. Hence, the altered bands are C_1^{*E} and C_4^{*E}. The coefficients of sub-bands produced are

$$\left[c_1^{LL_E^*} C_1^{LH_E^*} C_1^{HL_E^*} C_1^{HH_E^*} \right] = DWT(C_1^{*E}) \tag{14.10}$$

$$\left[c_4^{LL_E^*} C_4^{LH_E^*} C_4^{HL_E^*} C_4^{HH_E^*} \right] = DWT(C_4^{*E}) \tag{14.11}$$

The simulation outcome is

$$S_q^* = C_1^{K_E^*} - C_1^K; 1 \le q \le 4 \tag{14.12}$$

$$S_P^* = C_4^{K_E^*} - C_4^K; 5 \le p \le 8 \tag{14.13}$$

where $K = \{LL, LH, HL, HH\}, C_1^{K_E^*}$ is referred as coefficients of sub-bands of C_1^{*E}, C_1^K means sub-band coefficient of cover image, $C_4^{K_E^*}$ depicts the coefficients of modified sub-band C_4^{*E} of SI, and C_4^K denotes the sub-band coefficient. The SI is present in a binary form and it is binary. Also, decimal transformation steps and sparse signal are produced in decimal conversion. The obtained message is S^{*s}.

$$S^{*s} = \frac{S_{1 \times N}^{*d}}{S_{N \times N}^R} \tag{14.14}$$

where $S_{N \times N}^R$ implies a randomly produced sparse matrix and $S_{1 \times N}^{*d}$ represents a decimally transformed sparse signal generated from SI.

14.2.3 IPSO-BASED PIXEL SELECTION PROCESS

Here, the optimal location of a pixel is identified by the IPSO method. The CF is to estimate the fitness of all pixel positions. The projected CF is based on intensity, entropy, and the edge of single seed points of chromosomes. IPSO is defined as a stochastic optimizing method depending upon the population. It processes the initialization by the arbitrary collection of particles and explores optimal solutions under the position update of every particle.

It is considered that the swarm population is comprised of M particles in D dimensional space, and the historical optimal position of the jth particle is shown by $p_i, i \in \{1, 2, \cdots, M\}$, and the optimal location of the swarm population is presented as p_g. At each evolution phase, the velocity v_i and position x_i for every particle is upgraded by the observation of adjacent optimum position. In the case of fundamental PSO, control variables are composed with the performance of a model. When it is allocated ineffectively, the trajectories of particles cannot converge, which might be unstable, leading to an optimizing solution in optimizing issues. Recently, the control parameters are often selected based on experiments from scientists, because they are not stable and the searching facility of PSO is limited. The flowchart of IPSO algorithm is shown in Fig. 14.3.

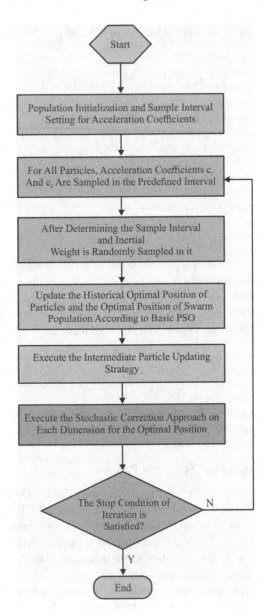

FIGURE 14.3 Flowchart of the IPSO algorithm.

A random sampling principle is developed to enhance the flexibility of control parameters and boost the searching potential of PSO to assist the jump out of local optima. Based on the convergence of PSO, the parameters are selected randomly. Initially, acceleration coefficients c_1 and c_2 are sampled uniformly in value interval, and parameters μ and σ could be estimated under the application. The condition of mean squares convergence as the sampling interval for inertial weight ω could be resolved

$$\underline{\omega} \le \omega \le \overline{\omega} \tag{14.15}$$

where $\underline{\omega}$ and $\overline{\omega}$, implies the lower and upper bound

$$\underline{\omega} = \frac{\mu^2 - \sigma^2 - \sqrt{(\mu^2 - \sigma^2)^2 - 8\mu((\mu-1)^2 + \sigma^2 - 1)}}{4\mu} \tag{14.16}$$

$$\overline{\omega} = \frac{\mu^2 - \sigma^2 + \sqrt{(\mu^2 - \sigma^2)^2 - 8\mu((\mu-1)^2 + \sigma^2 - 1)}}{4\mu} \tag{14.17}$$

Consequently, the inertial weight undergoes sampling with estimated interval. To eliminate the phenomenon of oscillation and two steps forward, one step back of inertia weight can be chosen at the center part of the convergence interval of ω. If the acceleration coefficients undergo sampling as $c_1 = c_2 = 2$, and parameters μ and σ^2 are evaluated, $\mu = 2, \sigma^2 = \frac{2}{3}$. The convergence of inertial weight is [0.333, 0.5].

According to the random sampling principle of every particle in swarm, upgrade the positions and velocity in all evolution phases. On the other hand, the intermediate particle updating strategy is devised to eliminate the primary randomness of sampling strategy in control parameters, and employed for upgrading the optimal location of the swarm population in all evolution steps. The technique to produce intermediate particles are provided as follows:

1. Intermediate particle 1 $(X_{iTemp}(1))$: the position of a particle in every dimension is average value of each updated particle in a similar dimension.

$$X_{itemp}(1)_d = \frac{\sum_{i=1}^{M} x_{i,d}}{M}; d \in \{1, 2, \cdots, D\} \tag{14.18}$$

2. Intermediate particle 2 $(X_{iTemp}(2))$: the rate of this particle in all dimensions is similar to the median of particles at the corresponding dimension.

$$X_{iTemp}(2)_d = median\ (x_{:,d}); d \in \{1, 2, \cdots, D\} \tag{14.19}$$

3. Intermediate particle 3 $(X_{itemp}(3)_d)$: every dimension value of a particle is one that is composed with a higher absolute value of high and low values.

$$X_{itemp}(3)_d = \begin{cases} \min(x_d) \mid \min(x_{:,d}) \mid > \mid \max(x_{:,d}) \mid \\ max\ (x_d) else; \end{cases} \tag{14.20}$$

$$d \in \{1, 2, \cdots, D\}$$

4. Intermediate particle 4 ($X_{iTemp}(4)_d$): All dimension values of a particle that has a minimum absolute value of maximum and minimum from adjacent dimensions.

$$X_{itemp}(4)_d = \begin{cases} min\ (x_d)\ |\ min\ (X_{:,d})\ |<|\ max\ (X_{:,d})\ | \\ max\ (x_d)\ else; \end{cases}$$

$$d \in \{1, 2, \cdots, D\}$$

(14.21)

Here, it is selected with optimal fitness value from for intermediate particles. When it has an optimal solution, the best position of the swarm population would be replaced; otherwise, it remains without any modification.

14.3 PERFORMANCE VALIDATION

The experimental assessment of the presented IPSO-DWT model takes place using a set of images. Fig. 14.4 shows some of the sample test images including Lena, Vegetable, medical images, and so on.

Table 14.1 and Figs. 14.5–14.6 show the results analysis of the IPSO-DWT model in terms of PSNR and structural similarity (SSIM). On applied image I1, it is exhibited that the IPSO-DWT model reaches a maximum PSNR and SSIM of 48.98 dB and 0.984, respectively. On applied image I2, it is exhibited that the IPSO-DWT model reaches a maximum PSNR and SSIM of 48.65dB and 0.973, respectively. On applied image I3, it is exhibited that the IPSO-DWT model reaches a maximum PSNR and SSIM of 45.20 dB and 0.993, respectively. On applied image I4, it is exhibited that the IPSO-DWT model reaches a maximum PSNR and SSIM of 46.23 dB and 0.995, respectively. On applied image I5, it is exhibited that the IPSO-DWT model reaches a maximum PSNR and SSIM of 46.37 dB and 0.986, respectively.

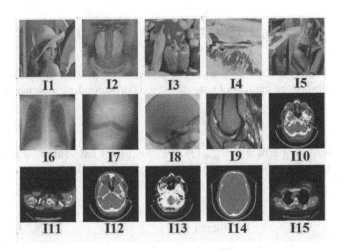

FIGURE 14.4 Sample test images.

TABLE 14.1

Perceptual Results Analysis of Proposed Method

Image Name	PSNR	SSIM
I1	48.98	0.984
I2	48.65	0.973
I3	45.20	0.993
I4	46.23	0.995
I5	46.37	0.986
I6	49.86	0.980
I7	45.08	0.981
I8	49.64	0.975
I9	46.30	0.996
I10	47.22	0.992
I11	46.31	0.984
I12	45.83	0.993
I13	46.21	0.994
I14	45.09	0.996
I15	46.54	0.985

In the same way, on applied image I6, it is exhibited that the IPSO-DWT model reaches a maximum PSNR and SSIM of 49.86 dB and 0.980, respectively. On applied image I7, it is exhibited that the IPSO-DWT model reaches a maximum PSNR and SSIM of 45.08 dB and 0.981, respectively. On applied image I8, it is exhibited that the IPSO-DWT model reaches a maximum PSNR and SSIM of 49.64 dB and 0.975, respectively.

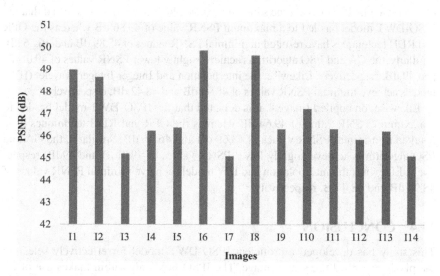

FIGURE 14.5 PSNR analysis of diverse models.

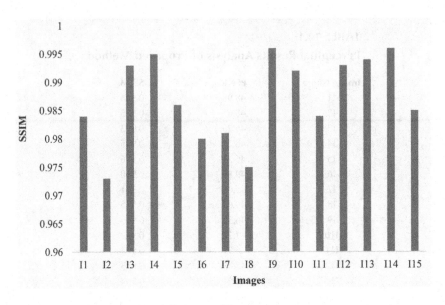

FIGURE 14.6 SSIM analysis of diverse models.

Table 14.2 shows a comparison of the results offered by the IPSO-DWT model with existing techniques in terms of PSNR. On applied Image 1, it is depicted that the IPSO-DWT model has led to a maximum PSNR value of 48.98 dB whereas the Optimal Pixel Repetition (OPR) and Reversible Data Hiding (RDH) techniques have resulted in minimal PSNR values of 43.88 dB and 46.36 dB. At the same time, on applied Image 2, it is depicted that the IPSO-DWT model has led to a maximum PSNR value of 48.65 dB whereas the OPR and RDH techniques have resulted in minimal PSNR values of 43.91 dB and 46.37 dB. At the same time, on applied Image 6, it is depicted that the IPSO-DWT model has led to a maximum PSNR value of 49.86 dB whereas the OPR and RDH techniques have resulted in minimal PSNR values of 43.89 dB and 46.36 dB. Similarly, the GA and PSO algorithms achieve slightly lower PSNR values of 49.01 dB and 49 dB, respectively. Likewise, the interpolation and Integer-Integer Wavelet (IIW) models achieve minimal PSNR values of 48.94 dB and 48.42 dB, respectively.

Likewise, on applied Image 8, it is depicted that the IPSO-DWT model has led to a maximum PSNR value of 49.64 dB whereas the OPR and RDH techniques have resulted in minimal PSNR values of 43.60 dB and 46.36 dB. Similarly, the GA and PSO algorithms achieve slightly lower PSNR values of 49.01dB and 49dB, respectively. Likewise, the interpolation and IIW models achieve minimal PSNR values of 48.94 dB and 48.4 dB, respectively.

14.4 CONCLUSION

This study has developed a proficient IPSO-DWT model for effectively selecting the pixels to embed the secret image. The IPSO-DWT algorithm makes use of FF with respect to CF. The CF evaluates the fitness based on the determination of the

TABLE 14.2
Results Analysis of IPSO-DWT with State-of-the-Art Methods

Image	Method	PSNR (dB)
Image 1	**IPSO-DWT**	**48.98**
	OPR	43.88
	RDH	46.36
Image 2	**IPSO-DWT**	**48.65**
	OPR	43.91
	RDH	46.37
Image 6	**IPSO-DWT**	**49.86**
	OPR	43.89
	RDH	46.36
	GA scheme	49.01
	PSO scheme	49.00
	Interpolation Technique	48.94
	Integer-Integer Wavelet (IIW)	48.42
Image 8	**IPSO-DWT**	**49.64**
	OPR	43.60
	RDH	46.36
	GA scheme	49.01
	PSO scheme	49.00
	Interpolation Technique	48.94
	IIW	48.42

edge, entropy, and pixel intensities to evaluate FF. An elaborate experimental analysis takes place to validate the goodness of the IPSO-DWT algorithm. The outcome ensured the optimal outcome of the IPSO-DWT algorithm in terms of SSIM and PSNR over compared methods. The experimental outcome stated that the IPSO-DWT model has resulted in maximal PSNR and SSIM models over compared methods in a considerable way. In the future, the IPSO-DWT model can be improved by the use of deep learning techniques.

REFERENCES

[1] Islam, S. R., Kwak, D., Kabir, M. H., Hossain, M., and Kwak, K. S. The Internet of Things for health care: A comprehensive survey, *IEEE Access*, 3, 678–708, 2015.
[2] Dimitrov, D. V. Medical internet of things and big data in healthcare, *Healthcare Informatics Research*, 22 (3), 156–163, 2016.
[3] Lakshmanaprabu, S. K., Mohanty, S. N., Krishnamoorthy, S., Uthayakumar, J., and Shankar, K. Online clinical decision support system using optimal deep neural networks, *Applied Soft Computing*, 81, 105487, 2019.
[4] Elhoseny, M., Bian, G. B., Lakshmanaprabu, S. K., Shankar, K., Singh, A. K., and Wu, W. Effective features to classify ovarian cancer data in Internet of Medical Things, *Computer Networks*, 159, 147–156, 2019.

[5] Kathiresan, S., Sait, A. R. W., Gupta, D., Lakshmanaprabu, S. K., Khanna, A., and Pandey, H. M. Automated detection and classification of fundus diabetic retinopathy images using synergic deep learning model, *Pattern Recognition Letters,* Vol. 133, 2020.

[6] Shankar, K., Perumal, E., and Vidhyavathi, R. M. Deep neural network with moth search optimization algorithm based detection and classification of diabetic retinopathy images, *SN Applied Sciences*, 2 (4), 1–10, 2020.

[7] Yang, H., Sun, X., and Sun, G. A high capacity image data hiding scheme using adaptive LSB substitution, *Radioengineering*, 18 (4), 509–516, 2009.

[8] Muhammad, K., Sajjad, M., and Baik, S. Dual-level security based cyclic18 steganographic method and its application for secure transmission of keyframes during wireless capsule endoscopy, *Journal of Medical Systems*, 40 (5) 114, 2016.

[9] Jung, K., Ha, K., and Yoo, K. Image data hiding method based on multi-pixel differencing and LSB substitution methods, in International Conference on Convergence and Hybrid Information Technology, 2008, 355–358.

[10] Muhammad, K., Ahmad, J., Rehman, N. U., Jan, Z., and Sajjad, M. CISSKA-LSB: color image steganography using stego key-directed adaptive LSB substitution method, *Multimedia Tools Applications*, 76 (6), 8597–8626, 2017.

[11] Chen, W., Chang, C., and Le, T. High payload steganography mechanism using hybrid edge detector, *Expert Systems with Applications*, 37 (4), 3292–3301, 2010.

[12] Muhammad, K., Sajjad, M., Mehmood, I., Rho, S., and Baik, S. A novel magic LSB substitution method (M-LSB-SM) using multi-level encryption and achromatic component of an image, *Multimedia Tools Applications*, 75 (22) 14867–14893, 2016.

[13] Laskar, S., and Hemachandran, K. High capacity data hiding using LSB steganography and encryption, *International Journal of Database Management Systems*, 4 (6) 57–68, 2012.

[14] Joo, J., Oh, T., Lee, H., and Lee, H. Adaptive steganographic method using the floor function with practical message formats, *International Journal of Innovative Computing, Information, and Control*, 7 (1), 161–175, 2011.

[15] Rahim, N., Ahmad, J., Muhammad, K., Sangaiah, A., and Baik, S. Privacy-preserving image retrieval for mobile devices with deep features on the cloud, *Computing Communications*, 127, 75–85, 2018.

[16] Chaumont, M., and Puech, W. A DCT-based data-hiding method to embed the color information in a JPEG grey level image, in 2006 14th European Signal Processing Conference, 2006, 1–5.

15 IoHT with Wearable Devices–Based Feature Extraction and a Deep Neural Networks Classification Model for Heart Disease Diagnosis

15.1 INTRODUCTION

Internet of Things (IoT) concepts are employed in diverse fields transforming the way that business processes are made [1]. Health informatics is a promising multidisciplinary domain that focuses on employing information engineering concepts to healthcare. The information usually originates from a diversity of sources such as healthcare information technology systems, but lately it is being saved in distinct IoT devices [2, 3]. The application of IoT concepts is becoming the norm, giving rise to the Internet of Health Things (IoHT). In general, heart disease (HD) is said to be a more serious disease that affects the function of the human heart and tends to increase the chance of a coronary artery or lower blood vessel event. Such complications lead to a heart attack or stroke. Based on the study of [1], around 610,000 people are affected by HD in the United States. Although HD affects males and females, males are more positive for heart attacks. The study reveals that the signs of HD [2] are chest tightness, pain, pressure, breathing issues, leg chills, neck pain, abdominal pain, tachycardia, light headedness, bradycardia, dizziness, syncope, change in skin color, leg swelling, weight loss, and fatigue. Sometimes, the symptoms differ based on the nature of HD such as arrhythmia, myocardia, heart attack, congenital HD, mitral regurgitation, and dilated cardiomyopathy. Some of the risk factors involved in HD are age, genetics, smoking, sex habits, drug abuse, higher cholesterol, high BP, external inactivity, obesity, diabetes, stress, and poor diet and hygiene. The severity of HD requires the disease analyzing process to be focused on diagnosing at an early stage.

While undergoing the screening process, physicians take into account the level of blood glucose, cholesterol test, BP test, electrocardiography (ECG), ultrasound, cardiac computer tomography (CT) calcium rate, and stress test. Therefore, the screening task [4] requires a massive time interval for manual intervention. There are various automated realizing models employed to find the function of human heart and pattern modification. Additionally, a few data mining (DM) methods, machine learning (ML), and artificial intelligence (AI) methodologies [5] were utilized to perform the heart information. For enhancing the model's function, an automated system extracts gathered data and removes the noise. Furthermore, diverse filtering approaches [6] such as normalization mean filters have been applied for processing the data [7]. Therefore, these automated models require a massive volume of data, which results in system complications. This difficulty tends to minimize efficiency in detecting HD. Hence, the automatic system is combined with a smarter device according to IoT [8] for collecting patient details.

Here, IoT is comprised of a set of devices and sensors that are employed to collect data from a specific platform. The efficiency of a sensor device was developed by Kevin Ashton at MIT campus. The tool applies the radio frequency ID and P and G sensor managing device [9] for gathering data from the human body. The Io- centric communication task [10] enhances the total experience of a patient and the common efficiency of this task. Here, the advantages of IoT devices are harnessed by combining with an automated disease detecting model for analyzing HD. At the time of processing this operation, the system might predict the HD features with minimum accuracy because it has poor training, learning, and examining processes. Hence, major contributions of this method are applied for improvising HD prediction value under the application of a massive amount of data, lower time consumption at the time of detecting HD, and assuring reduced false classification value during the detection of HD.

Broad research has been carried out for incrementing the diagnosis of HD. In [11], cardiovascular HD has been forecasted with the help of an optimized genetic algorithm (GA) with fuzzy recurrent network. Also, it is employed with a benchmark database to estimate the HD. The patient data is computed by applying data processing methodologies along with fuzzy-rule based technique. The recurrent network segments that provide input detects the attained results for effective training, which can be accomplished by using GA. Even though the developed model attains maximum recognition value, which tends to the production design of fuzzy classification rules, it does not provide exact accuracy for a massive amount of heart data. In [12], optimal neural networks (NN) were employed for finding HD-based information. It helps collect different clinical as well as heart data, which is computed successfully to remove the noise. Consequently, to diagnose the variations in data, it is provided into feed forward NN (FFNN). While processing the analyzing task, the parameters undergo optimization under the application of genetic operators, which reduce analyzing difficulty. Therefore, it is effectively deploying a method that predicts HD with maximum accuracy than conventional classification models like support vector machine (SVM) and k-nearest neighbor (K-NN).

In [13], the swarm optimized convolution neural network (CNN), with SVM, is applied in recognizing HD. While implementing, the deviation in a kidney, a test has been carried out under the application of chronic disease-based data such as saliva, ammonia, and concentration of urea. The data is computed using SVM along with a swarm intelligence (SI) training model. Furthermore, the affected features undergo classification by applying CNN, which analyzes HD with maximum accuracy.

Therefore, failure explains the efficiency of the feature selection (FS) process that produces the difficulty and improves the processing duration.

In [14], the efficiency of different intelligent health care modules, such as data transmission framework IoT, big data, and smart decision-making processes that are applied in disease diagnosis, is discussed. The gathered data undergo investigation by employing various ML techniques, stochastic models, and evolutionary approaches. The combination of these models leads to automated disease analysis for improving the total diagnostic process. Besides, even though it is applied in diagnosing diseases like diabetes and HD, it has failed to mention the way of capturing data from a subject, and tends to maintain the data analyzing process.

In [15], an IoT-centric HD recognition module is deployed based on the ML technique. The collected data has been computed with the application of SVM, which accurately classifies normal as well as a cardiovascular disease with higher accuracy. Therefore, the model collects details about HD such as body temperature, BP, heartbeat, and humidity level using IoT devices. It is repeated for obtaining accurate values regarding HD. Also, it is capable of recognizing HD with reduced time but fails to control the real-time heart data in the case of a higher amount of data in a technique. In [16], HD has been detected by employing the Cleveland clinic database with the help of particle-optimized feed forward back propagated NN (BPNN). The gathered features are examined based on selecting optimal features to particle position as well as velocity. Such features can be determined under the application of feed forward BPNN to attain the accurate features for abnormal HD. This method analyzes the HD with higher accuracy and reduced cost.

In [17], mortal HD predicting is deployed by using a particle swarm-optimized radial basis function network. The authors also look at HD details that analyze the heart features concerning nonlinearity as well as linearity. Also, extracted features have been computed, and selected features from abnormal HD features undergo classification. Hence, it is based on heart rate inter-beat (RR) interval to examine heart value with partial accuracy. Therefore, diverse automated models are capable of analyzing HD, but it requires a larger amount of heart details to improve accuracy. The newly presented method is applied for analyzing deviations in heart features with lower complexity as well as higher accuracy.

This chapter presents a new IoT wearable–based heart disease diagnosis model. The proposed model gathers the patient details and transmits the data to the health care center. Then, the feature process takes place followed by a deep neural network (DNN)–based classification. The proposed model will effectively predict the presence of heart disease from the data gathered by the IoT wearable. The effectiveness of the proposed model has been tested using a benchmark data set. The results indicated that the proposed model outperforms the existing models in a significant way.

15.2 PROPOSED MODEL

Fig. 15.1 shows the working principle of the feature extraction based DNN (FEDNN) model. In the beginning, the data collection process takes place followed by preprocessing. Then, the preprocessed data undergo feature extraction and extracted

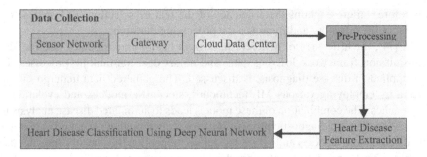

FIGURE 15.1   Overall process of proposed FEDNN.

useful features. Followed by, DNN based classification process takes place, which is explained in the following subsections.

15.2.1   IoHT-Based Patient Data Collection

Here, a HD detecting method is deployed with the help of the HOBDBNN model. The prediction method is combined with IoT, due to the presence of the automated system needing more amounts of patient data to improve the detecting accuracy. If the IoT device is located on the human body, it gathers data such as ECG, heart rate, BP, peripheral pulse oximetry (SpO2) level, glucose level, blood fat level, and pulse rate details. Hence, the collected data is converted to an alternate tool from a cloud database to monitor the patient's heart status. The IoT device and collated data have a portable watch to track the data about a patient using an IoT device.

The device is applicable in gathering a patient's heart value and saves external activities since the physical activities give suitable data about a patient's heart status; which is again provided to the health care center by Bluetooth links.

Here, IoT medical data is gathered under the placement of the sensor device on a human body. While the collected data is forwarded through the gateway and recorded in a cloud server. From the cloud, HD details can be forwarded in three major phases: heart data pre-processing, feature extraction, and HD prediction. The model cannot apply the FS algorithm because it is filled to predict HD by computing data and features. By analyzing these features, the executed system forecasts HD effectively to attain efficient training as well as classifiers.

15.2.2   IoHT Medical Data Preprocessing

The first phase in IoT is medical data preprocessing, which involves removing noise and missing data from the gathered information. Hence, noise-free data leads to an efficient analysis of HD derived patterns. Here, irregular data is removed under the application of the median studentized residual method due to the appropriate examina-tion of data from a data set, to improve the entire HD realizing task. At the initial stage, data is investigated using rows and columns, while missing values are interchanged by the evaluation of the median value. It is computed by arranging in improved order, while the center value is estimated. The median value has been employed because of the skewed minimum as well as outliers across the mean value. Under the application of center value, irregular values might be interchanged. Once the missing values are replaced, data should undergo normalization from the range of 0 to 1 to reduce the difficulty, thereby realizing HD patterns. Normalization is carried out with the help of several distributions of regression analysis of heart details. Moreover, data has been effectively normalized from the range of (0,1). Once the noise has been removed, diverse HD features are filtered for accurately classifying HD patterns.

15.2.3 HEART FEATURE EXTRACTION

The alternate step is to filter diverse features from IoT-centric medical details. The data set encloses data such as heart rate, BP, and blood glucose level. In order to attain the condition of HD, it is evident to obtain major features such as statistical and temporal features. The components of feature derivation are shown by the given equations

$$Peak\ amplitude = max\left(amplitude\ in\ stochastic\ period\right) \tag{15.1}$$

$$Total\ hormonic\ distortion = \frac{\sum all\ hormonic\ components}{power\ of\ fundamenfal\ frequency} \tag{15.2}$$

$$Heart\ rate = \frac{60}{RR\ Interval} \tag{15.3}$$

$$Zero\ crossing\ rate = sign\ change\ of\ signal\ (positive\ to\ negative) \tag{15.4}$$

$$Entropy = \sum_{ij=0}^{n1} - ln\ (P_{ii})P_{ii} \tag{15.5}$$

$$Energy = \sum_{ij=0}^{n1}(P_{ii})^2 \tag{15.6}$$

$$standard\ deviation = \frac{1}{N}\sqrt{\sum_{i=2}^{N}(RR_i - RR_{i1} - \mu)^2} \tag{15.7}$$

where RR is referred to as the interval of attained data.

$$\mu = \frac{\sum_{i=2}^{N}(RR_i - RR_{i1})}{N-1} \tag{15.8}$$

N denotes the overall count of RR intervals in data. Here, the root mean square of the sum of successive differences (RMSSD) is displayed

$$= \sqrt{\frac{\sum_{i=2}^{N}(RR_i - RR_{i-1})^2}{N-1}} \tag{15.9}$$

where N is shown as count of features, RR refers to the intervalue of heartbeat, μ implies mean value, and P_{ij} depicts the probability rate. Hence, the given features are obtained from data gathered from wearable IoT medical devices. It is provisioned as determinants to predict HD and modifies the HD pattern.

15.2.4 DNN FOR DATA CLASSIFICATION

Initially, it was evolved from the features of deep networks, named as a DNN-based approach with stacked autoencoders (SAE) for diabetes data classification that enhances every evaluation parameters of a classification issue. The DNN classification in the case of the diabetes data set is developed with the application of SAE as well as the softmax layer as defined. The data set is comprised of eight attributes and a class variable. These eight attributes are provided as input for the input layer. The DNN built contains layers of SAE. The network is composed of two hidden layers with 20 neurons. The softmax layer has the final hidden layer to perform classification performance. The output layer provides probabilities of diabetic as well as a nondiabetic classes for the provided data. Parameters employed for the developed model are provided in Table 15.1 and the architecture is shown in Fig. 15.2.

15.2.4.1 Training of Layers

Suppose N input vectors applied for training AE might be $\{x_{(1)}, x_{(2)} \ldots \ldots x_{(N)}\}$. The reformation of input is experimented by training AE as provided in the following:

$$x' = f_D(W', b'; f_E(W, b; x)) \tag{15.10}$$

This can be written

$$x' = f_{AE}(W, b, W', b'; x) \tag{15.11}$$

where f_{AE} is a function that maps input to output in AE.

TABLE 15.1

Sensitivity Analysis of Existing with Proposed FEDNN Method

Methods	Number of Patients				
	500	750	1,000	1,250	1,500
GA-TRFNN	94.24	95.04	95.48	96.43	96.89
SCNN-SVM	95.23	95.78	96.30	96.87	97.20
PFFBPNN	96.35	96.82	97.02	97.48	97.87
PSRBFN	98.21	98.35	98.54	98.76	98.89
FEDNN	98.54	98.78	99.13	99.16	99.32

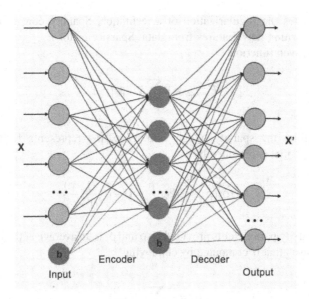

FIGURE 15.2 DNN architecture.

Here, AE could be trained by reducing the proper objective function that is providing overall error function as

$$E_{Total} = E_{MSE} + E_{Reg} + E_{sparsity} \qquad (15.12)$$

where $E_{MSE}, E_{Reg}, E_{sparsity}$ are mean squared error, regularizing, as well as sparsity factor, correspondingly. The mean squared error, E_{MSE} could be estimated by

$$E_{MSE} = \frac{1}{N} \sum_{i=1}^{N} e_i^2 \qquad (15.13)$$

where e_i denotes the error, that is a difference among actual output, $x(i)$ and the monitored output, $x'(i)$. The error e_i might be determined as

$$e_i = \left\| x(i) - x'(i) \right\| \qquad (15.14)$$

Deep networks understand each point from the training data set, which leads to overfitting of the technique. It is referred to as a problem along with deep networks since it offers poor performance based on novel testing data. For resolving the problem, regularizing factor, E_{Reg} is assumed in an objective function that is estimated by applying

$$E_{Reg} = \frac{\lambda}{2} \left(\sum_{i=1}^{c} \| w_i \| + \sum_{i=1}^{D} \| w_i' \| \right) \qquad (15.15)$$

where λ denotes the regularization of a technique. Sparsity constraint enables a method for learning new features from data. Sparsity factor $E_{sparsity}$ is estimated by applying the given function

$$E_{sparsity} = \beta \sum_{i=1}^{c} KL(\rho \| \rho_j) \qquad (15.16)$$

where β implies the sparsity weight and $KL(\rho \| \rho_j)$ represents KullbackLeibler divergence[1λ–λ3] that is provided by

$$KL(\rho \| \rho_j) = \rho log \frac{\rho}{\rho_j} + (1-\rho) \frac{(1-\rho)}{(1-\rho_j)} \qquad (15.17)$$

where the sparsity parameter is provided by ρ and ρ_j is an average activation measure of the jth neuron that is computed by employing

$$\rho_j = \frac{1}{T} \sum_{i=1}^{T} f^j(x_{(i)}) \qquad (15.18)$$

where $f^j(x_{(i)})$ is an activation function of the jth neuron.

15.2.4.2 The Stacked Autoencoder

A deep network that applies AE has been developed by cascading the encoder layers as given in Fig. 15.3. Recall that the mapping of AE from SAE is shown as

$$f_{SAE} = f_E^1 \circ f_E^2 \circ f_E^3 \dots \circ f_E^L \qquad (15.19)$$

where the SAE function is given as f_{SAE}. For every layer of SAE, the encoder function is employed. It is more significant that the decoding function is not used for every layer.

15.2.4.3 The Softmax Layer

Softmax classification is said to be a multiclass classifier that uses LR to classify the data. The softmax layer employs a supervised learning model that utilizes upgraded LR for classifying several classes. Hence, LR is based on the softmax classifier. In the case of multiple classification issues, the softmax classifier calculates the probability of every class where it performs data classification. Therefore, the sum of probability is 1. The softmax function performs the normalization and exponentiation

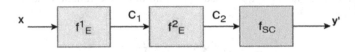

FIGURE 15.3 Stacked autoencoder with L layers.

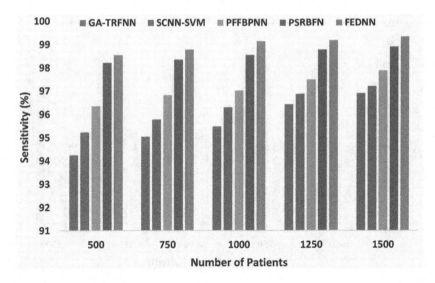

FIGURE 15.4   Sensitivity analysis.

that are used to find the class probabilities. Hence, the softmax layer with function f_{SC} is embedded with SAE.

15.3   PERFORMANCE VALIDATION

The results attained by the FEDNN method have been tested under diverse scenarios. Fig. 15.4 and Table 15.1 depict the sensitivity analysis of diverse models under a varying number of patients. The table values indicate that the FEDNN method achieves maximum sensitivity under all patient scenarios. Under the existence of 500 patients, it is noted that the FEDNN method leads to a maximum sensitivity of 98.54% whereas the GA-TRFNN, SCNN-SVM, PFFBPNN, and PSRBFN models reach slightly lower sensitivity values of 94.24%, 95.23%, 96.35%, and 98.21%, correspondingly. Under the existence of 750 patients, it is noted that the FEDNN method leads to a maximum sensitivity of 98.78% whereas the GA-TRFNN, SCNN-SVM, PFFBPNN, and PSRBFN models reach slightly lower sensitivity values of 95.04%, 95.78%, 96.82%, and 98.35%, correspondingly. Under the existence of 1,000 patients, it is noted that the FEDNN method leads to a maximum sensitivity of 99.13% whereas the GA-TRFNN, SCNN-SVM, PFFBPNN, and PSRBFN models reach slightly lower sensitivity values of 95.48%, 96.30%, 97.02%, and 98.54%, correspondingly. Under the existence of 1,250 patients, it is noted that the FEDNN method leads to a maximum sensitivity of 99.16% whereas the GA-TRFNN, SCNN-SVM, PFFBPNN, and PSRBFN models reach slightly lower sensitivity values of 96.43%, 96.87%, 97.48%, and 98.76%, correspondingly. Under the existence of 1,500 patients, it is noted that the FEDNN method leads to a maximum sensitivity of 99.32% whereas the GA-TRFNN, SCNN-SVM, PFFBPNN, and PSRBFN models reach slightly lower sensitivity values of 96.89%, 97.20%, 97.87%, and 98.89%w correspondingly.

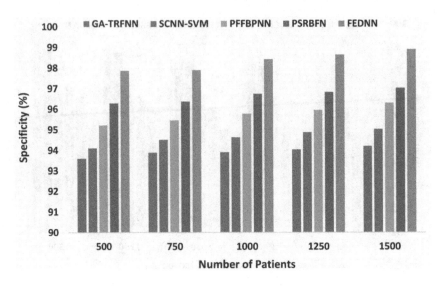

FIGURE 15.5   Specificity analysis.

Fig. 15.5 demonstrates the specificity analysis of diverse models under vary-ing number of patients. Table 15.2 values indicate that the FEDNN method achieves maximum specificity under all patient scenarios. Under the existence of 500 patients, it is noted that the FEDNN method leads to a maximum specificity of 97.87% whereas the GA-TRFNN, SCNN-SVM, PFFBPNN, and PSRBFN models reach slightly lower specificity values of 93.60%, 94.10%, 95.21%, and 96.28%, correspondingly. Under the existence of 750 patients, it is noted that the FEDNN method leads to a maximum specificity of 97.90% whereas the GA-TRFNN, SCNN-SVM, PFFBPNN, and PSRBFN models reach slightly lower specific-ity values of 93.89%, 94.52%, 95.46%, and 96.37%, correspondingly. Under the existence of 1,000 patients, it is noted that the FEDNN method leads to a maxi-mum specificity of 98.43% whereas the GA-TRFNN, SCNN-SVM, PFFBPNN, and PSRBFN models reach slightly lower specificity values of 93.91%, 94.63%, 95.78%, and 96.74%, correspondingly. Under the existence of 1,250 patients, it is

TABLE 15.2
Specificity Analysis of Existing with Proposed FEDNN Method

	Number of Patients				
Methods	500	750	1000	1250	1500
GA-TRFNN	93.60	93.89	93.91	94.04	94.21
SCNN-SVM	94.10	94.52	94.63	94.87	95.03
PFFBPNN	95.21	95.46	95.78	95.95	96.30
PSRBFN	96.28	96.37	96.74	96.82	97.02
FEDNN	97.87	97.90	98.43	98.65	98.91

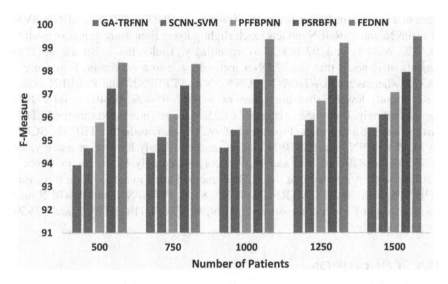

FIGURE 15.6 F-measure analysis of various models.

noted that the FEDNN method leads to a maximum specificity of 98.65% whereas the GA-TRFNN, SCNN-SVM, PFFBPNN, and PSRBFN models reach slightly lower specificity values of 94.04%, 94.87%, 95.95%, and 96.82%, correspondingly. Under the existence of 1,500 patients, it is noted that the FEDNN method leads to a maximum specificity of 98.91% whereas the GA-TRFNN, SCNN-SVM, PFFBPNN, and PSRBFN models reach slightly lower specificity values of 94.21%, 95.03%, 96.30%, and 97.02%, correspondingly.

Fig. 15.6 depicts the F-measure analysis of diverse models under a varying number of patients. Table 15.3 values indicate that the FEDNN method achieves maximum F-measure under all patient scenarios. Under the existence of 500 patients, it is noted that the FEDNN method leads to a maximum F-measure of 98.37% whereas the GA-TRFNN, SCNN-SVM, PFFBPNN, and PSRBFN models reach slightly lower F-measure values of 93.92%, 94.66%, 95.78%, and 97.24%, correspondingly. Under the existence of 750 patients, it is noted that the FEDNN method

TABLE 15.3
F-Measure Analysis of Existing with Proposed FEDNN Method

Methods	Number of Patients				
	500	750	1,000	1,250	1,500
GA-TRFNN	93.92	94.46	94.69	95.23	95.55
SCNN-SVM	94.66	95.15	95.46	95.87	96.11
PFFBPNN	95.78	96.14	96.40	96.71	97.08
PSRBFN	97.24	97.36	97.64	97.79	97.95
FEDNN	98.37	98.30	99.37	99.21	99.48

leads to a maximum F-measure of 98.30% whereas the GA-TRFNN, SCNN-SVM, PFFBPNN, and PSRBFN models reach slightly lower F-measure values of 94.46%, 95.15%, 96.14%, and 97.36%, correspondingly. Under the existence of 1,000 patients, it is noted that the FEDNN method leads to a maximum F-measure of 99.37% whereas the GA-TRFNN, SCNN-SVM, PFFBPNN, and PSRBFN models reach slightly lower F-measure values of 94.69%, 95.46%, 96.40%, and 97.64%, correspondingly. Under the existence of 1,250 patients, it is noted that the FEDNN method leads to a maximum F-measure of 99.21% whereas the GA-TRFNN, SCNN-SVM, PFFBPNN, and PSRBFN models reaches slightly lower F-measure values of 95.23%, 95.87%, 96.71%, and 97.79%, correspondingly. Under the existence of 1,500 patients, it is noted that the FEDNN method leads to a maximum F-measure of 99.48% whereas the GA-TRFNN, SCNN-SVM, PFFBPNN, and PSRBFN models reach slightly lower F-measure values of 95.55%, 96.11%, 97.08%, and 97.95%, correspondingly.

15.4 CONCLUSION

This chapter has introduced an effective IoT wearable–based HD diagnosis model. The proposed model gathers the patient details and transmits the data to the health care center. Then, the feature process takes place followed by DNN-based classification. The proposed model will effectively predict the presence of heart disease from the data gathered by the IoT wearable. The effectiveness of the proposed model has been tested using a benchmark data set. The results indicate that the proposed model outperforms existing models in a significant way. The experimental outcome pointed out that the proposed model reaches maximum sensitivity, specificity, and F-score. In the future, the performance of the proposed model can be further enhanced by the use of diverse clustering techniques.

REFERENCES

[1] Ansari, S., Aslam, T., Poncela, J., Otero, P. and Ansari, A., Internet of Things-Based healthcare applications, in *IoT Architectures, Models, and Platforms for Smart City Applications*, IGI Global. 2020, 1–28.

[2] Darwish, A., Hassanien, A.E., Elhoseny, M., Sangaiah, A. K. and Muhammad, K., The impact of the hybrid platform of internet of things and cloud computing on healthcare systems: opportunities, challenges, and open problems, *Journal of Ambient Intelligence and Humanized Computing*, 10 (10), 4151–4166, 2019.

[3] Challoner, A. and Popescu, G.H., Intelligent sensing technology, smart healthcare services, and internet of medical things-based diagnosis, *American Journal of Medical Research*, 6 (1), 13–18, 2019.

[4] Elhoseny, M., Shankar, K., and Uthayakumar, J. Intelligent diagnostic prediction and classification system for chronic kidney disease, *Scientific Reports*, 9 (1), 1–14, 2019.

[5] Lakshmanaprabu, S. K., Mohanty, S. N., Krishnamoorthy, S., Uthayakumar, J., and Shankar, K. Online clinical decision support system using optimal deep neural networks, *Applied Soft Computing*, 81, 105487, 2019.

[6] Elhoseny, M., Bian, G. B., Lakshmanaprabu, S. K., Shankar, K., Singh, A. K., and Wu, W. Effective features to classify ovarian cancer data in internet of medical things, *Computer Networks*, 159, 147–156, 2019.

[7] Shankar, K., Perumal, E., and Vidhyavathi, R. M. Deep neural network with moth search optimization algorithm based detection and classification of diabetic retinopathy images, *SN Applied Sciences*, 2 (4), 1–10, 2020.

[8] Raj, R. J. S., Shobana, S. J., Pustokhina, I. V., Pustokhin, D. A., Gupta, D., and Shankar, K. Optimal feature selection-based medical image classification using deep learning model in Internet of Medical Things, *IEEE Access*, 8, 58006–58017, 2020.

[9] Ashton, K. That 'Internet of Things' thing, *RFID Journal*, 22, 97–114, 2009.

[10] Alarifi, A. and Tolba, A. Optimizing the network energy of cloud assisted internet of things by using the adaptive neural learning approach in wireless sensor networks, *Computers in Industry*, 106 133–141, 2019.

[11] Uyar, K., and Ilhan, A. Diagnosis of heart disease using genetic algorithm based trained recurrent fuzzy neural networks, *Procedia Computing Science*, 120 588–593, 2017.

[12] Chitra, R., and Seenivasagam, V. Knowledge discovery from heart disease dataset using optimized neural network, in R. Prasath, T. Kathirvalavakumar (Eds.), *Mining Intelligence and Knowledge Exploration*, Springer, Cham, 2013.

[13] Navaneeth, B., and Suchetha, M. PSO optimized 1-D CNN-SVM architecture for real-time detection and classification applications, *Computers in Biology and Medicine*, 108, 85–92, 2019.

[14] Chui, K. T., Alhalabi, W., Pang, S. S. H., Ordóñez de Pablos, P., Liu, R. W., and Zhao, M. Disease diagnosis in smart healthcare: Innovation technologies and applications, *Sustainability,* 9, 2309, 2017.

[15] Ahmed, F. An Internet of Things (IoT) application for predicting the quantity of future heart attack patients, *IJCA*, 164 (6) 36–40, 2017.

[16] Nashif, S., Raihan, Md. R., Islam, Md. R., and Imam, M. H. Heart disease detection by using machine learning algorithms and a real-time cardiovascular health monitoring system, *World Journal of Engineering Technology*, 6, 854–873, 2018.

[17] Feshki, M. J., and Shijani, O. S. Improving the heart disease diagnosis by evolutionary algorithm of PSO and feed forward neural network, Artificial Intelligence and Robotics (IRANOPEN), 2016.

Index

Italicized and **bold** pages refer to figures and tables respectively

Printed in the United States
by Baker & Taylor Publisher Services